# Successful to Burnt Ou
# Autistic Women

By Karletta Abianac

Featuring contributions by Lorraine Abbott, Kathy Isaacs, Laina Eartharcher, and Liz Marxon

The circumstances and conversations are recalled to the best of the author's ability. Errors are purely unintentional.

Second Edition. Updated 2019

Successful to Burnt Out: Experiences of Autistic women / Karletta Abianac; contributions by Lorraine Abbott, Kathy Isaacs, Laina Eartharcher, Liz Marxon

Print Edition ISBN-13 978-1-925955-03-3
eBook Edition ISBN 13 978-1-925955-04-0

BIO033000  BIOGRAPHY & AUTOBIOGRAPHY / People with Disabilities
BIO022000  BIOGRAPHY & AUTOBIOGRAPHY / Women

Cover page image by Cherry Penman, 2015. Used with permission.

Dedicated to the adult actually-Autistic bloggers and advocates.

*"Nothing about us without us."*

This memoir explores my story of Autistic burn out, and includes experiences of four other Autistic women (Autism Spectrum, Asperger's, an Aspie).

This second edition now includes relevant blog posts written and published on Musings of KarlettaA. You'll find Karletta's musings on masking, mental health, burnout and recovery, goals, and the profound power of silence when overwhelmed.

Successful to Burnt Out features women who've considered ourselves successful in our primary role. We've had to slow down or stop working.
Some of us didn't know why life became exponentially harder. Why we had burnt out.
We realised our limitations and finally put names to them. Anxiety. Depression. Late in life, we found out it was also from being on the Autism Spectrum.

How have we dealt with being a shell of what we once were?
How did we go from being successful to burnt out?
Where are we now in life's journey?

This book is the first in the 'I've been there too Darl' Autism memoir series.

You can keep updated on my writing and provide feedback on future books through my email list at http://eepurl.com/cBDCmH

# Chapter One: Being Successful

## My Achievements

I imagined that by the time I hit twenty-five, I'd be working full-time in a job that I loved. It turned out that I was an independent contractor working on community projects occasionally.

I was struggling but considered myself successful.
I had received an award from the Queensland Government and spoken at events to a couple of hundred people.
I was an emerging Community Cultural Development worker, Public Speaker, and Workshop Facilitator.
I had written and released an eBook in 2004 on community event management. Years earlier I had occasionally published a street magazine. As it turns out, my articles were written for young people on the Autism Spectrum (Asperger's, an Aspie). My favourite articles were on renting your first house and on managing your budget.

Things I'd achieve would bring me back to happiness and pride. My accomplishments gave me a purpose and self-identity if I concentrated hard enough. And I did have to concentrate to feel purposeful.

## Contributing to Society

After a Business Administration Traineeship, I completed a mentor program in 2004, being mentored, through Youth Arts Queensland. The program was called Young Artists Mentor Program.
During the program, I had learned more about festival management and drawing on the wisdom of local community groups. I was working at the time with the Visible Ink Youth Festival, for the second year in a row. Visible Ink is, among other things, a hub for young people to run business and projects. It is part of or funded by, Brisbane City Council.

I wrote an eBook about Community Event Management for my end of year project. I eagerly project planned and wrote, with the idea of sharing printable templates and practical advice. This came from hearing of frustrations of some of the contractors and volunteers. Each year they would have to create the documents from scratch. I saw a vacancy of a book and ran with it.
The eBook was called Fill in the Gaps. It was distributed on CD ROM and later on a couple of websites. The Visible Ink program paid for the layout to be redone by a graphic designer. At this time the designer renamed the document to Filling in the Gaps. I've got to admit, I never quite took to that title. I was referring to the actions of writing on printed templates.

Sometime in 2003 I became emotionally heavily invested in a personal development company. The company was big on the concept of transformation. At times I would completely alter my experiences of life and my identity. These changes would be huge. There seemed to be no room for changing yourself in small increments.
I liked to think that by volunteering for the company, I was helping people deal with their problems. I felt like I was contributing to the wellbeing of society. Helping friends and families reconnect. It felt like I was helping people have an easier, more manageable life.

I took on two public speaking courses back to back, and refined skills that helped me create better speeches and be calmer on stage. Before getting involved in the company, I had done five to ten-minute spots here and there. I've spoken at program launches, conferences and as part of a panel. I felt useful and valued during those commitments. After doing the public speaking courses, I facilitated at a conference and ran a few workshops.

## Identity

I think that your sense of identity is something that gets confirmed and created in conversation. In a way, it can be something held outside of you. This identity exists without you needing to remember it. A friend said to me in 2015 'I remember you as a workaholic'. I felt a sense of peace and identity from her saying that.

Back in the years when I was emerging in the youth community sector, I used my accomplishments to explain my identity. When I needed a sense of self, which was often, I imagined myself at work and volunteering. Whether it was things I'd done, wanted to do or even imagining how I was making a difference to someone I'd met.

An award I got in 2003 summed up my life purpose well. The Youth Up Front Award from the Queensland Government was for my "commitment to social change and volunteer efforts". That's what the minister Matt Foley said in his congratulations letter. Well, the one he signed anyway.

During the period of 2001-2007, I tried to keep myself as busy as I could but was often still on the Dole (Newstart Allowance). Sometimes I felt like a fraud. Here I was on the Dole, yet also contributing, in my mind, to society. As you can imagine, there were many internal conflicts.

## Internal Conflicts

I frequently felt nervous and uncomfortable for no reason, yet at times created a sense of calm and stillness when on a stage speaking to an audience.

I couldn't get rid of my doubts, nervousness, and awkwardness for long, yet at times could create an all-encompassing way of being. For instance: being loving, being compassionate, being purposeful, being willing to fail and being committed.

The moments in time that I relished above all, were being determined, peaceful and compassionate. Inevitably, however, I'd 'wake up' in a few days or hours. No motivation would be left to make myself continue a task I was doing. I felt a range of emotions from weirdly uncomfortable up to distressed.

I could be productive and successful for short stretches of a time, then suddenly be worn out. This had many manifestations. I called them my unproductive side. I couldn't concentrate, was fed up and easily frustrated, and at times couldn't make myself work. I was becoming unreliable at finishing a task or project. At times eager and willing to work on something for days straight, then utterly unmotivated.

*DSM 5 Diagnostic Criteria B.3.*

*Highly restricted, fixated interests that are abnormal in intensity or focus (e.g, strong attachment to or preoccupation with unusual objects, excessively circumscribed or perseverative interest).*

Weirdly I felt like someone was always aware of what I was doing. It could have felt like a flat mate in another part of the house, people around me while standing in line or even in the privacy of my own lounge room. I wondered if this was psychosis or paranoia. It turns out to be linked to a lack of Theory of Mind (ToM). It is where you can't separate your point of view with someone else's.

At times I was bubbly and open with my speech. Then there were times when I couldn't explain my work, disagree with someone's assumptions of my work or flat out didn't know what to say next. I felt 'held back' from speaking. I assumed that I couldn't have a communication problem because I was articulate, both in spoken and written words. In fact, having learned apparently exclusive communication skills through the personal development company, I felt that I had exceptional skills in this area.

## A Common Experience

I could be convinced that everyone had it this hard. I'd hear ableist sayings like 'No one likes their job' and 'everyone has bad days'. When I could hear myself making a fool of myself or being embarrassingly awkward, I just assumed it was part of learning and growing as a professional.

I kept going about things as usual, with many strategies for pushing away or accepting my unproductive side. The strategies included these things, which I wrote in my public speaking eBook. The section was on managing how you are in the present. There are times on a stage when thoughts pop up, and you just had to dismiss them.
What did I have to say about dealing with feelings and thoughts? 'Ignore them, give up the right to feel that way, let go of thoughts, drop them and don't believe them'. There was 'give yourself no-room to concentrate on anything but the audience receiving a clear communication.' I would 'Imagine an empty space after the moment of the thought. Fill it with what you intend to achieve out of your speech'.
Being present, or in the moment was a tool I often used, for many years, both on and off stage. The practical side of me loved the space where I'd 'acknowledge to yourself that nothing has changed in the physical universe. What matters now is delivering your speech well'. In life, I started to laugh at people who'd call me names. Their words were utterly disconnected to me. Meaningless. 'You don't have to think about anything for more than a second' was helpful, except when the feelings would come around time and time again. Like endless ocean waves.

I learned to develop a sense of compassion for myself. In lieu of a boyfriend, at times I would imagine that I was loving and caring to myself. This was quite a nice experience, but I would have loved to felt it from another person!

Forgiveness was something I had to create often. I wasn't working as often as I knew I could. I was given all sorts of *sarcasm alert* helpful advice; 'You just need confidence', 'you've got to try harder', 'you've just got to put yourself out there' and my favourite 'You just need to finish things'.

All very useful for someone, maybe, but if those things were relevant; I knew they were shallow solutions.

## Explanations

I was always trying to explain and get to the source of why I got unproductive and held back from speaking. What stopped me from finishing a project?

I developed explanations for my unproductive side. Oh, I was uncomfortable? I must be confronted by something. Feel like some things missing? Mate, it's a human experience all through life. Nervous and weak tongued? Surely I've just not said something to someone or owe them an apology. Frustrated, off balance and upset you say? Must be upset because something expected or intended didn't pan out.

In short, I was left with the impression (that sometimes negatively persists today) that there was an optional way of explaining and dealing with my unproductive characteristics. I could or should take responsibility for these actions. This was both a blessing and a curse.
I could take responsibility and feel ownership and freedom that that could bring. The downside was managing my feelings from one minute to the next. When managing the thoughts and feelings worked it was great. When it didn't work, I felt burdened and confused. I mean, why would something work before but not now?

## On Fire

I could see the finished product of being productive and working full-time, but couldn't readily access it.

To paraphrase a previous employer, when you're good, you're on fire. When you're bad you're a disaster.

How could I be on fire one moment and a disaster the next day?

How could I be productive one minute and unproductive half an hour later?

# Success Contributions

## By Rae, A Community Nurse Specialist

I was a single mum with three children. Age thirty-one, I put myself through a year of college and then went to University to train as a nurse for three years. I found the course relatively easy and came out with a BSc Hons (2:1)
I got a job as a community nurse – I was good at it, and I really loved it.

Two years later, I was invited to interview for specialist training to become a qualified District Nurse. I was successful and went back (to a different) university to do a Masters level program to gain the community specialist practitioner qualification.
I did the V150 prescribing course and became a community nurse prescriber, undertaking specialist training in palliative care, leg ulcers and also in communication.

With my qualifications, I easily got a higher paid job. But never really had the confidence – always thinking the other staff knew better than me because most of them had been qualified longer. I had some time off work with 'depression' due to being in an emotionally abusive relationship, and looking back also possibly also due to strain/pressure I put on myself to be 1000% at all times.

When I went back (to a new team) I felt like I had lost all my skills and confidence. So, I moved jobs – essentially with a promised promotion to a sister of the hospital – but the job was given to a nurse with little experience.
My next job was a specialist role – but I quickly became bored and didn't feel my skills were being utilised. I looked for a new job and got a job as a trainee lecturer back at my original university – which was what I had always wanted: 'my dream job'.

## Kathy, Owner of Access Health Autism

After school, I did a Bachelor of Science but didn't want to work in the field I'd studied, so I puttered about looking for something to do and landed in Aged Care via volunteer work. I really enjoyed the interaction with residents, so I decided to study, and was able to complete my Bachelor of Nursing in 2 years, thanks to my Science degree.

I enjoyed nursing and was accepted into my first preference for a graduate year, being given two interesting and challenging rotations in oncology. From there, I found my true home in community palliative care. The chance to make a difference, to help people through my increasing knowledge and my ability to see patterns; gaining a firm grounding on what really matters in life – these times were precious.
I started honours immediately after I'd finished my graduate year. Although I completed the coursework with top marks, I withdrew from the thesis when I got pregnant.

After our son was born, I maintained part-time work while my husband studied nursing. I had undiagnosed post-natal depression, but I still managed to juggle work and the baby as well as read over my husband's essays and assignments. Home life was a grey blur for two years, but I could still bracket the depression for a time in order to function, and the haze cleared after two years.

After my second child was born, two and a half years later, I started a Masters in Palliative Care. Whilst doing this, I worked in community palliative care. I supported and advocated for my son through school and the process of chasing a diagnosis. We had a house designed and started to move towards having it built. I also started edging into the academic world by presenting posters and small talks at national conferences.

## Laina, An Integrative Medicine Doctor

I don't know if I would call myself "successful", at least by Neurotypical society's standards), but other than my chronic indecision about what I ultimately wanted to do with my life, I was holding it together.

I was going to university and changed university majors 8 times. To support myself I worked anywhere from 10-45 hours a week as a cocktail waitress.
I had been able to fake it while waitressing. Mainly because I didn't really have a choice (we desperately needed my income). While still drifting between majors, I burned out of waitressing. It was something that we (my partner and I) had to deal with. It happened sooner than we could afford.

## Liz, A Musician

My career was in the music industry. I was a leader in my field for the greater part of my twenty-year career. I have many releases in Australia and overseas. I have chosen to write under a pseudonym here, as I am still going through my own process of self-discovery and acceptance. I used to tour across Australia and occasionally internationally.

Music was my whole life. It's all I talked about, and all I did. Looking back, I must have driven people crazy. When I was at home, I was writing music, I have a degree in music, when I went out at night it was to hear the music I loved, to try and get gigs (at first) and to work. All my friends worked in the industry either as musicians, disc jockeys, video artists, or photographers. The latest releases were all we talked about.

I have auditory sensitivities and I could hear things in music that no one else could. At the start I had to do everything the right way, as I saw it, for example, getting a Bachelor of Music, so I could be confident and knowledgeable. I also did a business course and received a grant to launch my own business. Having the degree and the business training gave me confidence in trying to get gigs and releases with record labels. I was also a woman in the boys club that was the music industry at that time. There was only a sprinkling of females in the industry, although this has changed now.

I am proud of my career achievements, and I'm lucky to have had many females starting their careers call me their inspiration, which for that, I am honoured.

# Chapter Two: Slowing Down

## Uncomfortable

When I signed up for a public self-development seminar, I was hoping to slow down or stop my numerous thoughts.

After filling out their paperwork, in which you were required to tell them if you had any mental health problems, I didn't think that childhood and teenage depression would be an issue. I'd got myself over that. The only concern I had I shared with a friend. In the conference room, before it started, I told her I was worried that bad memories would stay with me long afterward. She assured me that it would be fine. I took her at her word.

After a few months, for something to do, I offered to volunteer with them. The introductory meeting inspired me a lot. Taking my self-development seriously, I attended and volunteered at a lot of seminars for the company.

I am glad that I went to the seminars because I learned over the years to take responsibility and many other life skills. However, I was very impressionable. I took things literally. I felt I had an exciting obligation to attend more and more.

As I said before, I created different personifications and feelings of myself. Ways of Being they were called. However sometimes within a day of a feeling naturally dissolving, I would feel unusual. I couldn't describe it much at the time. If I asked for coaching, the conversations might be circular, with no resolution. A couple of coaches told me that I was wasting their time. Still, I was never supported when I told people that I wanted to take a break. There is a concept they use where you realise that other people are afraid of looking like a fool in front of you. 'So that's why I'm nervous all the time' I thought.

I learned to like myself. I practiced being compassionate and loving to myself. Be the parents I wished I'd had. Relaxed into enjoying my own company.

I could believe that people loved me, liked me, or respected me. Or just reveled in knowing that people's feelings were nothing to do with me. I learned how to exude my interest in a person's feelings. Lost myself in each moment. Returned to me again. I meditated. Took my time doing things well. Was content.

Over the years, however, the nervousness would not let up. I was feeling uncomfortable a lot more than other people seemed to be. I tried many times to tell my coaches 'I don't feel right'. The people I spoke to would refuse to consider that I was experiencing anything they didn't themselves. I went through cycles of feeling on fire, and then wanting to take a break. The people I spoke to would always insist I not listen to my reasons for quitting. 'Be unreasonable' was frequently banded around.

Thinking positively, and feeling that I had nothing to lose, I applied for and got a job opportunity for the company. I was really excited. I was finally going to get paid for making a difference to people's lives!
It required a move in 2005 to Sydney, NSW, Australia. Rushing around, getting ready for the move, my flat mates told me I was worrying too much about certain things. One thing they mentioned, but I dismissed, is that I took things literally. On a call from Sydney, I was told in an offhand or motivational remark to not come down until I had somewhere to live. I was frantic for a week, anxiously trying to find accommodation, dreading not being able to work for this company that I loved. In the days prior to getting on the plane, I kept leaving phone messages that went unanswered, asking if I should still come down. I hadn't found accommodation.

## Frantic and Nervous

I was on Reception at their busy office. Their phones ran off the hook and I could not answer all the calls. Frequently four to six phone lines would be busy or be ringing at once. If I was supposed to enlist volunteers to help, I failed.

I didn't know it then, but I have trouble communicating with people. Being tongue-tied, nervous and overwhelmed is not a good thing for someone on reception. The only words I had for this at the time were 'nervous' and 'I can't keep up'.

I felt so guilty putting someone on hold the minute I answered. Only a few times did I handle all the calls well. That was over a four-month period.

In 2005 I was fired or quit for not doing my job. In any case, I told my boss I was worried about my wellbeing. (Wellbeing was a term used in the company I was with. It was, as I understand, a reference to people who couldn't do their seminars due to mental health issues. You have to vet yourself on whether you can handle the 11-hour seminars and philosophical content.)

I was asked to stay until they'd found a replacement. That last month was a kind of living hell.

Being fired was both a mighty relief and utter disappointment. I say fired but, yes, I know I raised the possibility of leaving. It felt like being fired. Back in Brisbane, I nursed my injured pride for failing what I felt should have been an easy job. I also came back with a take no nonsense attitude that had been wonderfully heightened in Sydney. My blunt speech had been honed into pure direct honesty.

## Slowing Down

Back in Brisbane, Queensland I limited my parameters for working. 'maybe not a full-time job just now. Go back to temporary work.' I knew I was burnt out.

Inexplicably I was experiencing increasing flashes of frustration, anger, and feeling trapped while working even week-long assignments. These didn't make sense, so I began thinking there was still something wrong with my wellbeing. My mental state just wasn't settling down.

I began what would become years of interviews and sessions with mental health nurses, psychologists, psychiatrists, and doctors. I discovered things that started to make sense of my unproductive side. I had anxiety. My mind was blown. My depression was back. Bugger. I have schizo affective disorder. Excuse me?
What I explained as a vivid imagination combined with anxiety was now called paranoia. Imagining conversations to combat loneliness was psychosis. Streaks of productivity were mania. 'Isn't that just called working?' I thought.

A psychiatrist helped a shocked yours truly to get on the Disability Pension. I further reduced my temporary jobs to a day or two here and there. Emergency relief. Thank god I didn't have to deal with the fear and crushing obligation of having to look for work every week. I hated looking for work, partly because I never got past the interview stage. I was thoroughly sick of going to interviews and never getting a job.
At the time I didn't know any unwritten rules. I didn't (and still don't) see the point in wearing makeup, and had no concept of the social and personal boundaries I was crossing. In short, I had no idea of what people might think of me, and the many ways people judge others. Just what an interviewer wants.

I didn't realise until years later that while I'm articulate, I also have a communication disorder. I didn't even know that those two things could co-exist.

*DSM 5 Diagnostic Criteria A.3.*

*Deficits in developing, maintaining, and understanding relationships, ranging, for example, from difficulties adjusting behavior to suit various social contexts; to difficulties in sharing imaginative play or in making friends; to absence of interest in peers.*

## Missing Hidden Contexts

For an example of how a lack of social skills can play out at work, I'll take you back to one temporary job in Brisbane City.

I got a call from a lady I knew in a temporary work agency. She offered me a job which I repeatedly tried to turn down. I was volunteering that night and had a lot of phone calls to make, plus knew I'd have to leave early. It didn't occur to me to tell her my reasons for why I couldn't accept the job assignment. That is a lack of Theory of Mind right there. I thought that saying 'I can't-do it' was enough information for her. It would have been for me. Finally, out of exasperation and feeling backed into a corner I agreed. There was, unfortunately, a proviso not communicated on my part. If they were going to take my time away from volunteer work at home, then they can pay for my time. I would make the calls at work. Again, it didn't occur to me that she needed to know these feelings. Surely, I thought, she can hear my reluctance. She knew I had things to manage.

During one of the phone calls, two ladies from the workplace stood near me, talking.
I looked over at them a number of times, but they seemed to return my looks blankly. I asked if they'd like a tea or coffee, it being part of my job to make them. They declined a drink. I didn't know why they were standing there, as to me there was no sign of wanting me for anything. Maybe they just wanted a change of scenery.
Unknown to all of us, I was not able to read their body language, the situational contexts or their facial expressions. If I had, they would have been telling me something like:

We want to talk to you.
We want you off the phone.
Making personal calls is not acceptable.
If I did suspect that they wanted me off the phone, I assume I would have dismissed it thinking 'You made me come in. Now let me do my actual job.'
I do know that I felt trapped that day. Like I couldn't leave but I had to do my volunteer work as well.

The feedback from the job was bad, and rightly so. I must have embarrassed the recruitment lady, who I had known personally. When I accepted that temp assignment, I didn't know that I listen to the content of what people say only. I didn't understand that there is a whole lot of communication that is not in physical reality. I'm talking the contexts, assumptions, situational contexts and reasons behind what people say. People not on the Spectrum (Neurotypicals) need to know the reasons and contexts for things. Saying 'I can't-do it' wasn't good enough. People don't seem to take you at your word.

**Anxiety**

Examples like this, of times I acted inappropriately at work, made my career stressed all my life.

A lot of conversations - no matter how short - were fraught with hidden traps to stumble into. An example of this is the character Clayton Bigsby, in Dave Chapelle's sketch program, Chappelle's Show. Clayton is blind, in the KKK, and doesn't know he is an African American. I was talking blindly.
As you may imagine, simply leaving the house was to enter another potential situation of misunderstandings and nervousness.

At that point, I couldn't identify what made me nervous. In an effort to explain it, misplaced anxiety had me fearing a roof would blow away in a storm, or, as had happened at school, that someone would punch me at random.

I just thought I was unlucky and got an Anxiety gene in fetus development.


## Fired Again

I think I stopped working even temporary jobs the day I was fired from a recruitment agency. All morning I had been trying to force myself to leave the house but was unable to make myself get on the bus to a job.

Once again it was a relief to not have to force myself to leave the house, but it was also a shock. 'I should be working full time' I kept telling myself.

By 2006 I finished volunteer work for the self-development company. I was constantly feeling awkward, on display and very uncomfortable. A little bit of being uncomfortable is to be expected. This happens when you go outside of your comfort zone. The level of these feelings, their constant, repetitive nature was not. I was having wild mood swings. Having to manage my feelings minute to minute was exhausting. I knew this wasn't normal, although, being a personal development company, people tried extremely hard to tell me that what I was feeling was normal.


## Self Employed

Trying out being a self-employed workshop facilitator, I ran three workshops in 2005.

The workshops were on Community Project Management, Reviewing and Planning for New Years, and on Branding Yourself as an independent arts worker. The workshops had less than five people attend each, which was both disappointing and exciting. I knew I was starting out as a workshop facilitator and could expect low numbers. I was also excited because people actually came to them!

Taking my self-employment very seriously, I kept myself busy with business administration. I'd written a business plan, marketing plan, and five workshops. I'd also designed various business forms and templates in Microsoft Word.

# Slowing Down Contributions

## Kathy

Juggling all of these responsibilities (my son's diagnosis, house design, working and studying) I found that I was dissociating from worrying about them by bracketing anxiety in my mind – the same technique I used when dealing with depression.

At the 'business end' of my Masters in October 2014, with a major project to hand in, grappling with the Council over their delay in approving our house plans, juggling appointments for my older son who wasn't coping at school.
Hardest of all was staying with a friend while we waited for the house to be built, who hadn't realised my kids really are different from "normal" kids. He didn't seem to like them very much.
The stress became too much and I took leave from work, two weeks of sick leave, and two weeks of annual leave. By the end of November, with the Masters completed, the house underway, things felt settled.

However, in the middle of the next year, 2015, it became clear that my anxiety and depression hadn't been a reaction, and hadn't gone away with the improvement of my situation. My stress levels rose again and I tried to rationalize them away, but one day at work, it was like something cracked inside me, and I could no longer ignore or rationalise it.
I called in sick, took myself off the roster for another two weeks, and sought help from my GP. I started antidepressant medication and some counseling. I found that my work environment was no longer supportive, and my manager advised me that he had seen me struggling with my mental health, and had known that I was "going to let [him] down". This stunned me and caused the 'crack' to break completely.

Despite returning to work for a while, I was despondent, felt irrelevant, and resigned from permanent work six months later.

## Laina

During my time as a cocktail waitress, I knew I was burning out; it set in gradually, but it was undeniable.
I dreaded every shift and I was relieved when I had days off. I felt a huge disconnect, as I was moving more towards a healthier lifestyle, and yet my job and its environment embodied all things unhealthy. The divide grew wider and wider.

Finally, one day, I was fired. My ego felt a little bruised; I had always been the one to leave my previous jobs, and I had usually done so in good standing. But this time I had no warning; I was just erased from the next week's schedule. Part of me was shocked; the other wasn't. The latter part of me saw it coming and knew that it was just a matter of time.
I also panicked; we were barely making our monthly bills as it was. I called my partner at work and told him what happened. Luckily, he was very supportive and he cheered me up.
Still shaken by the sudden change of plans, I headed home fairly quickly and began that day to research the idea of becoming a massage therapist. I had been considering the idea before that, and I knew I was going to have to leave that job in about 4 months anyway, in order to go to school. But the bottom fell out from under me a little early.

The most comfortable financial state was during the massage therapy years. As I was reaching my peak, I was able to feast for a little while on a decent income, and we were finally able to get caught up on our bills. One would think that "Hey, I'm a doc now. I've hit the big time!" But not quite. In fact, I almost burned out during my first year in practice!

## Liz

Although I was totally happy with my career choice, there were factors that made me extremely anxious or overwhelmed. Touring takes its toll on you in so many ways. Physically it is exhausting, there are weekends that I'd work at night time and travel during the day, sometimes all day, to get to the next gig. It is very isolating, I would travel alone, be in hotels alone, and never have down time to recover. I didn't have a manager, although I did have a booking agent for a while.

I had to manage every aspect of my career, as well as be the creative. So organising tours, releases, media, and press. In fact, writing and producing music is about 10% of the job. Dealing with the industry while managing my career was extremely exhausting and difficult for me. Talking about music was lovely, but when dealing with the business side I was a mess, and although on the exterior I was composed and reserved, my insides were always in fight or flight mode.
I used to have to write down what I was going to say before making a phone call and make sure I had recovery time after a weekend of touring. I usually wouldn't surface until Wednesdays after a weekend. So, Mondays and Tuesdays were phone days. And then it would start over again.

# Chapter Three: Autistic Burn Out

## Burn Out

Referring to Maslow's hierarchy of needs, I knew that a number of things in my life were not working well. I didn't have stable accommodation. Due to my anxiety, I often felt fearful. I was not eating well, sometimes one or two meals a day.

I lacked confidence in handling my emotions, and situations at work, at home, and with my finances. My immediate future seemed bleak. I hoped that one day, in the next couple of years maybe, I'd be working full-time again. It just didn't seem possible then and there.

I tried to keep myself busy with writing poems and reading. I wanted to volunteer a few days a week but was living out past Sunnybank, an outer suburb of Brisbane. Getting to know new people and blending into a new community seemed a huge set of challenges.

## Unstable Housing

At about 2007 I was still having trouble finding stable housing. I wasn't a very good flatmate. When it came to clean most things, particularly the bathroom, I would feel nauseous, dirty and repulsed. This was due to the smells and also my vivid imagination came into play. My brain would shoot up vivid videos of dirty water being absorbed into my flesh.

*DSM 5 Diagnostic Criteria B.4.*

*Hyper- or hyporeactivity to sensory input or unusual interests in sensory aspects of the environment (e.g., apparent indifference to pain/temperature, adverse response to specific sounds or textures, excessive smelling or touching of objects, visual fascination with lights or movement).*

As you can imagine, I avoided cleaning as much as possible. This was especially true when it came to cleaning a house to get our bond back. Thoughts of days and days of cleaning were enough to overwhelm me and make me retreat to my room, shuddering under the bed covers.

Finding a new house was fraught with its own challenges. Think traveling, finances, interviews, and references.

There was the nervousness and strange tingling sensations whenever I had to catch a bus, to find a house where I was being interviewed. I found out later that this comes down to not being able to deal with a change of scenery very well. I couldn't deal with a change of routine very well either.

*DSM 5 Diagnostic Criteria B.2.*

*Insistence on sameness, inflexible adherence to routines, or ritualized patterns or verbal-nonverbal behavior (e.g., extreme distress at small changes, difficulties with transitions, rigid thinking patterns, greeting rituals, need to take same route or eat food every day).*

Interviews were wracked with tension. This is if I ever got to the interview stage of course. In one share-house website that I joined, I must have sent off messages to twenty houses, registering my interest. I got a call or message back from three and found one that was kind of suitable. Often, I'd move into places desperate for somewhere to sleep that week.
I can imagine that I missed a lot of hidden meanings in the interview questions and answers. I was taking people's words literally. I thought that adding meaning to what people were saying was called making assumptions. To assume was to 'make an ass out of you and me'. I had been humiliated enough in my life. To assume hidden meanings would heap more social embarrassment on me when the scenario turned bad.

I learned not to apply for share house adverts with the words fun, party or social. I was experiencing social exhaustion without having a name for it. Nowadays, years after my diagnosis of Autism Spectrum (Asperger's), I know that one hour of socialising requires two to three hours of recovery in a dim, quiet room. Then I can come out and do some chores. Sometimes even then I can only do a little random socialising for the rest of the day.

I thought of myself as a professional independent contractor. In reality, I was on the Disability Pension and rarely working. I was volunteering a couple of days a week but had no independent income. I was a homebody with lots of ideas that I sometimes spent hours writing down.

This created tensions in some housing. I was seen as lazy and not trying hard enough.  As one home owner-occupier said 'If I knew you weren't working, I wouldn't have had you here'.

That shocked me to my core. Why am I having to constantly prove myself to flatmates? Like, really? Do you not see who I am? Are you not listening?

## Financial Challenges

Being on the Dole (Newstart Allowance, then Disability Pension) meant I either couldn't afford to live in really nice houses or was rejected during interviews. People wouldn't trust that I could afford rent. In some ways they were right. On time, certainly. Especially when it came to leaving the house to get cash.

I needed the security of Centrepay to pay my rent on time. Centrepay in Australia is where Centrelink pay your selected bills before they pay you the Dole. I relied on Centrepay because I was far too impulsive for my own good. My bank offers a Christmas Club account, where if you take money out before November, they charge fifteen dollars per transaction. When I was impulsive and anxious to have money, that fifteen-dollar fee would mean nothing to me.

## Uncertain

I was frequently worried about being kicked out of my current housing. It was hard to live in one place for more than a year or two.

I had the conflict resolution skills of a much younger person. Any serious discussions about cleaning, rent, and visitors were filled with apprehension of being kicked out.

Usually, I left in a bad way. I was running away from confrontations or possible arguments. This meant that I didn't have any references until I was about thirty-two.

 I was always hesitant giving names and numbers for references in any case. I felt like I couldn't write my friends down, who I'd known for years, simply because they'd be biased towards me. Surely a real estate agent wouldn't want bias?

At times when I was desperate for somewhere to live the next week, I didn't approach the Department of Housing for help. My name had been on a list for years. I thought 'If they haven't found me one yet, there isn't one available.' I didn't understand about their priority levels of assessing people's needs.
I thought simply that potentially being homeless next week wasn't the same as living on the streets. Therefore, I couldn't be a priority. Therefore, there still isn't a house available for me.

## A Change

In the midst of one of these times of not being able to find a new share-house, I asked my mum if I could live with her for a few weeks. She lived in Rockhampton, Queensland which required a flight up from Brisbane. I only intended to stay there for a few weeks while looking for a good share house.

I stayed in that area for three years.

## Crashing

Within two months of moving in with my mum, I had crashed. I was a shell of who I once was. The change had been fast and devastating.

I shut down. It was like depression without sadness. It was being exhausted. Not giving up – but my mind and body just saying "Nope".

It was weird. In some ways, I regressed to a teenager. I was experiencing life as I used to back then. Feeling stuck, trapped, helpless and hopeless. Like nothing I had done to better myself had worked. Not in the long term anyway. I still relied on other people's goodwill for somewhere to live. I hadn't had a full-time job in years. I still didn't have a boyfriend. I still experienced Anxiety and Depression.

Surely with years of being involved in a personal development company, I would have changed more. Didn't I do rigorous self-development work while learning to lead their basic seminars? Surely that would have meant my life should be drastically different.

*DSM 5 Diagnostic Criteria C.*

*Symptoms must be present in the early developmental period (but may not become fully manifest until social demands exceed limited capacities, or may be masked by learned strategies in later life).*

## Disparity

The disparity between my vision of what I knew I was capable of, and what I was actually doing, was vast. I felt it like a yawning chasm.

I knew my worth. Knew how valuable it is to be vulnerable, compassionate, and share moments of tenderness. Not just moments, but spaces in time. Seeing through people's words to their beautiful souls.

I was told once that I was a friend who is easy to be around. I try to be accepting, peaceful, attentive with my friends. I also have a great memory for conversations, which I hoped people liked.

I learned to show up when people need to be heard. Be present. Be with them at that moment. Silently feeling with them. Being still and peaceful in our own little bubble.

To further expand on who I thought I was, and what I was capable of, I was a small business manager, contribution to society, an ideas person, entrepreneur, volunteer, committee member and public speaker. I hoped I was well regarded for my skills in project planning, public speaking and life coaching.

Why was I randomly going from productive to confused! Still. Not even a question. Just – this doesn't make sense.

How could I be confident, yet randomly go shy? Still. Even when it is vital to be my best. Even when ten minutes ago I was literally in the zone?

One incarnation of myself in the self-development days was being a Stunning Goddess. I tried to generate this in looks and demeanor. This is one of the deliberate ways I created a sense of self.

I had gone from this, to knowing I couldn't get through half a day of work, clean the kitchen or find a share-house. I felt useless, not taken seriously anymore. I felt guilty for being what others would call a dole bludger.

Something fundamental had said "Nope". I was like what...? I'm sorry, what just happened?

Since I had no business or community project news, I felt that I was no longer relevant to the community circles I formally worked in.

## Intentional

The times when I was working and productive in years past, I reveled in feeling intentional. I'd work with a clear a purpose for my actions. I remembered times of having a laser-like focus and concentrated thought processes.

I experienced this in 2009 while writing my eBook 'How you can BE an Amazing Public Speaker'.

From writing to promotion, it took about a week. That shows my lack of impulse control at the time. I needed to get that work out there. No time for a long editing process and significant rewrites. No letting it sit for a few weeks, unread.
I was following my own rules and being creatively free. So much so that it didn't have a devoted cover page, index or introduction section. The title was misleading. I had actually gone through myths of public speaking. It touched on views of how you could make room for intentionality and your natural voice.

Still, I was eagerly driven for a while. It was a blessed reminder that my productivity was still in there somewhere. That I would work again.

# Autistic Burn Out Contributions

## Rae

I loved the university environment. There was so much knowledge and expertise, and access to more at your fingertips.

But I hated being in a noisy office with three other people who were much more talkative/social than I was. I stopped going in early. I could work from home a lot - and did so as much as possible – too much. It began to feel alien going into work. Then I'd feel guilty for not going into work.
I started to feel panicky at what I was being asked to do – I was teaching people to become nurses but was losing all my confidence and clinical skills.
Organising my diary became problematic; I turned my work phone permanently onto voice mail and requested people to contact me by email whenever possible. I started avoiding things that caused me stress, and making excuses for not doing things. Even writing/typing became problematic and I started to wonder if I had developed dyslexia. Everyone else seemed to be doing well – but I felt like I was sinking, I felt like a fraud and I'm still not sure why.

Being in work, and doing a good job is important to me. It's not good enough for me to be a decent nurse/teacher – I have to be brilliant. I was in a constant state of emotional/tearful high alert with my fight or flight reflex permanently set to fly. I couldn't keep it up, and I couldn't see a workable way out.

Then somebody mentioned autism. I read a little, then booked myself on a conference – which felt like 'this is your life' – I could relate to everything they said so strongly. I took a couple of autism tests online and was off the scale. Went to see my GP, had a chat, and she referred me for assessment. I handed my notice in at work – the only viable option I could see.

I had the first part of the autism assessment last week. I had interviews lined up for nursing jobs – but I've cancelled them as I know I'm mentally not strong enough to get the jobs or cope with rejection. At the end of the month I will be unemployed.

## Laina

I started med school to get my physician's license, and opened my own practice nurturing it while it grew. Between school and setting up my practice, I burned out of massage therapy.

What I had is known as "physician burnout", which happens a lot; it's a commonly shared experience. It's when the effort you put forth outweighs the (positive) response/feedback from (or good progress by) patients for too long. I was working so hard, giving so much away, that was never appreciated. People might think "you're a doctor. First world problem. Hard to cultivate sympathy." And for many docs, that statement might be right. But we were actually living in a fairly low-income apartment because, well, our income was that low. We lived among gangs, drug dealers, and cockroaches for the first 2 years.

We didn't sign on with insurance companies because they get in the way of real patient care when it comes to chronic diseases, which was what I wanted to focus on because the conventional medical system usually fails these people so egregiously (I'm one of them). So, we weren't getting the referrals from those companies, nor those people who want or need to utilize their insurance.
Trying to do all of our own promotion and find those who didn't care about using their insurance is a very uphill struggle, and a very different income level than the docs who are part of The System.

I wrecked my joints, too, so that clinched it. Physical problems suddenly mushroomed. After a long road, I realized I was Celiac and neurologically messed up. There's a third time, a dang-near-burnout, in my current life as a doc.

**Liz**

At this point I did nothing to address my anxieties and some days, depression. In fact, I don't think I even recognised them for what they were.

I self-medicated with alcohol and other things. I refused to seek any help, let alone medicate for something like anxiety. I discovered alcohol. It proved an effective way for me to deal with the negative aspects of my career, and the fame, the anxiety and the social world around me. I was never addicted. I would never say I was an addict, in the traditional sense of the term. It is more the way that you would take prescribed medication, you take it, and it fixes the problems you are having. There is a massive problem with dealing with issues in this way. Ultimately, they make things worse.

I always wonder what life would have been like if I was diagnosed and knew why I was so affected by things other people didn't get affected by. Life was so draining and in the second half of my twenty-year career, things were taking their toll, physically and mentally. I had autoimmune health issues coming up more constantly. I was also taking longer to recover from my touring. I was disappearing out of the world more and more. I was burning out.

**Diagnosis**

My music career wound up around 2010, and my last gig was at the end of my second trimester. I was pregnant with my beautiful little boy.

He has changed my life forever. I am not going to go into specifics about him, but through his journey, I discovered the wonders of neurodiversity, and have only recently been diagnosed with Autism.

I am 42. I have been identifying as Autistic for about 2 years now. It has brought relief in so many ways, and a new light and understanding to who I am, who I was as a musician, and explained so many thoughts, actions, and behaviors.

I spend a lot of time reflecting on my career. I attribute all my strengths to being Autistic, including sensory sensitivities, incredible memory, the ability to see patterns in things and people, the ability to review legal documentation without a lawyer, being able to read a crowd – the list is endless.
There is a dark side though. And the only reason a dark side exists, for me, is because I went through my career as undiagnosed. The dark side isn't about Autism. It is about the mental illnesses that arise from spending my life in a constant state of anxiety, self-criticism, and blame.

# Chapter Four: Relevance Deprivation

## Irrelevant

Feeling irrelevant had a few entry points. Historically, I communicated with even my friends to pass on and receive information. I didn't know how to talk to them without news.

I didn't know how to hold a small talk conversation, other than to share news and useful information. My personal rule was no complaining and no gossiping. I was interested in social issues, personal growth, and running a small business.

I had no news about the Community Sector. No developments in my life, apart from business ideas and draft business plans.

Nothing to talk about.

*DSM 5 Diagnostic Criteria A.1.*

*Deficits in social-emotional reciprocity, ranging, for example, from abnormal social approach and failure of normal back-and-forth conversation; to reduced sharing of interests, emotions, or affect; to failure to initiate or respond to social interactions.*

I was unreliable so wouldn't commit to any projects or jobs. While living in Rockhampton, I couldn't participate in Brisbane based community events, where my friends and networks were.

I missed the times when I felt part of a movement. I missed those times when people were taking my advice. It seemed that my thoughts no longer mattered to anyone. I no longer felt valued. I missed times when people were relying on me to get something important done.

I felt relevance deprivation in the midst of unacknowledged Autistic Burn Out.

## Isolated

I felt separate from others in Rockhampton.

The working class didn't seem to have a very responsible work ethic. I couldn't respect someone when they left things to chance, with a 'that will do, it doesn't have to be perfect' attitude. I prefer to do everything I can at work, even if it's not necessary.

Feeling separate from the working class, the only friends I could make were pot smokers. Sometimes I could see them look at each other, aghast at what I'd said.
I was easy to manipulate, not being able to say no when they expected me to lend them some of my stashes. I learned to say no, but the persistent questioning and demanding would mean I'd hand some of it over more often that I liked.

I hated being addicted to pot, it being something else that made me feel trapped. It felt such a waste of money. The money I could have been saving up to move into a new house.
However, I smoked it because it would bring about a shift in my mental state. It also slowed down my thoughts, which were frequently racing by and being intrusive. Having smoked it, I could sometimes feel too exhausted to worry about anything.

## Humiliation

Normally in those days, I felt ashamed and separate from others from being unreliable and not working full-time. I was embarrassed that I was an adult living with my mum. I was frustrated that I couldn't find a long-term share-house.
I was also sure that when I was talking with people, my eyes looked like I was crazy. This explanation was what I used to justify having a hard time looking in people's eyes. I wondered if, in the past, the explanation was that feeling like a fraud held me back. These explanations didn't quite fit. I hoped there was a bigger picture explanation for why I seemed shy.

Because of my anxiety around cleaning, I tried to access home-support. I was knocked back with 'You don't need help around the home. No one likes cleaning.' And 'We can't support you because you don't have a severe disability.' Mum and I ended up hiring a regular cleaning service.

I'd think, or others would say to me that I'm leeching money out of government coffers. There is such a strong sense from some people that no self-respecting person would allow themselves to stay on the dole. I was told I should be working with phrases like 'Just get a job, you'll be great. You'll surprise yourself.', 'I don't know why you're on the dole' and 'No one likes working'.

I felt that I couldn't be respected because I'd succumbed to Depression and Anxiety. I felt that I couldn't be respected because I was on the Disability Pension. It was rare that I could concentrate while studying, which would improve future employment. I felt broken, with no way to regain my productivity. Even if I did gain my productivity and creativeness, I feared that I was too weak to follow through the project until the end. Therefore, I wouldn't commit to big projects or volunteer jobs.

## Cleaning Anxiety

One thing that I still have trouble with now days is making myself clean the house.

It takes a combination of things for me to be able to complete a cleaning task. First, I have to feel free to do it. As in, not dreading it, my body movements do what I want and I see a point to doing it. Not only do I have to see the point, but I have to grasp it and hold onto it. Holding onto a feeling of needing to do something is a huge challenge for me. I will either clean the house out of fear, from a clear feeling of wanting to do it or because someone has just told me they expect me to do it.

I must be annoying to live with, as I need constant reminders why something is important. As much as I logically know 'the dishes need cleaning', there is often a murkiness and anxiety there. Holding on to feeling why a task needs to be done is something I will be working on with my psychologist at some point.

I've also found that working on something gradually, every now and then, over time works best for me when I can't make myself do something then and there. In cleaning, I call it Spring Cleaning, as in the first breaths of spring air in a season.

## Dismissing my Diagnosis

In 2012 a Clinical Psychologist diagnosed me with being on the Autism Spectrum.
I don't have a clear memory of this, but it is possible he asked if I'd like him to explain about Asperger's. I would have laughed out a 'No'. Of course, I didn't have any form of Autism. It wasn't at all relevant to me. I could just imagine the shame of being referred to as a retard by others.

I don't know what I knew about the Autism Spectrum and Asperger's, but I did know that I was not confined to a wheelchair, unable to speak. Sure, I'd been unable to speak for the past six months. Only half-formed words would come out. Surely that would have been physical somehow. Even a physical examination showing nothing wrong didn't convince me. They must have missed something, surely!
Thinking of Louise Hays books on healing yourself, I thought maybe I couldn't speak because I didn't feel safe in speaking to my mum. She would share too much information about me to others.

I did a brief bit of research online about Asperger's but didn't relate to anything I read.

## Independence

I called the Department of Housing a couple of times to ask how my application for housing is going. On one conversation I asked that a couple of suburbs be changed from Brisbane to around Rockhampton. I was desperate to move into my own place. I didn't want to live with my mum anymore.

Unfortunately, that call finally triggered some action, because within two weeks I had been accepted for a house in a country town. I was angry at myself for changing my suburbs. That would turn out to be another two years of isolation, Depressive states, and continued Anxiety.

However, during those years in Mount Morgan, Queensland, I committed again to building my life from scratch. This time I practiced using a long-term outlook.

# Relevance Deprivation Contributions

## Kathy

In the time between returning to work the second time and resigning, I had an abstract accepted for a conference, one of only two from my organisation, and the only person asked to give a presentation, a 'speed-talk'.

Despite having been encouraged to pursue the project, the organisation later decided not to pay my conference registration. I paid for my own registration and used annual leave to attend. Seventeen people from my organisation were at the conference that day. While the speed-talks were well attended, none of them showed up except my project partner – and even she didn't stay for the whole presentation. This contrasted to the well-attended talks given by staff at previous conferences, and I felt gutted and rejected. After the conference, the Director and CEO advised me that they would not be supporting the project after all.

I felt that my strengths – research and presenting – were now utterly worthless to the organisation, and my weaknesses – socialising with colleagues and needing to work overtime to finish the day's work – were all that anyone ever saw. Despite still doing the core work of nursing professionally, I felt useless, worthless, and started to doubt my competence in that, too. I felt that I'd wasted my money and time doing the Masters; that it was a detriment rather than a benefit.

When I resigned from the permanent nursing role it seemed that my manager was relieved and glad to see me go.

This perception was confirmed two years later when, more emotionally stable, I applied for my old job, and he rejected the application, saying he believed I "might become unreliable again" due to my previous sick leave. He had also, as my primary referee, passed on these concerns to several potential employers, meaning I couldn't get any other work, either.

## Diagnosis

In January 2015, after my son's autism diagnosis, I was reading about the way's autism may present and laughing over a passage, "Denial and Arrogance", that read like a skillfully-worded description of both my father and my older son. When I read the next section, "Imitation", however, I stopped laughing because it described me. Although we'd always said Gareth was "just like me", what that meant hadn't sunk in until then.

I became obsessive in my reading, drawing on as many sources as I could – journals, autobiographies, blogs, textbooks, lectures and presentations, and the more I learned, the more I recognised myself. I threw myself into online autistic women's groups and found, for the first time in my life, that I didn't have to camouflage.
I was part of a tribe where people had similar struggles, similar stories, and really understood the daily labour involved in being autistic. My previously confusing personal history – a strange patchwork of extreme competence and sudden ineptitude; strongly held, immutable opinions and chameleon-like camouflage in groups – made coherent sense.

I began to feel internal pressure to seek a diagnosis. I wanted to be absorbed into this area but didn't feel I could say I was autistic if it was only my conviction underlying that.
Despite our reduced financial situation, my husband agreed that this was "something I had to do". Approaching the assessment, suddenly I was terrified that I'd be told I wasn't autistic. What if the only group that had ever understood me wasn't my "tribe" after all? When I went for the assessment results, I was visibly shaking. The psychologist understood - her first words to me were "Well, you're definitely Aspie". I was so relieved I actually whooped.
I felt free to start moving my work life into autism support and advocacy.

## Laina

I feel relevance deprivation on a fairly regular basis since starting practice, and I actually feel it most with some patients, surprisingly.

I had struggled through med school, but that was mostly internal. Interestingly enough, I had a sufficient number of friends in med school, and I got along with professors pretty well, too. My struggles mostly involved learning difficulties. I can learn quite efficiently when the material is presented in a particular manner, but it was presented in a manner that was incompatible with my learning style.

The relevance deprivation I have felt since graduation involves my own self-doubt about whether or not I actually feel appreciated by patients for the effort put forth on their behalf. I have experienced disrespect, irrationality, immaturity, false accusations (such as not having done something they wanted that I actually did, or having done something wrong that I actually didn't do, etc). Most of all, I'm tired of the bitching and complaining that I hear at times.

I know that it sounds like this happens all the time, but truthfully, it's actually a very small percentage of the time. However, as I'm sure you know, any "little" hiccup can cause major ripple effects for long periods of time in us Aspie/autistic peeps. And that's certainly true for me as well.

## Liz

When I wrapped up my career, I went into a state of mourning. It was everything to me, but I wasn't interested in pursuing a career anymore.

I was a mother now, and I tried to combine the two but it wasn't working. I wasn't self-medicating anymore and everything was bubbling to the surface. My anxiety was so high, coupled with a baby who did not sleep and my own insomnia, I was at breaking point. But I didn't have time to worry about me, and I became a mother who was obsessed with being perfect. Perfectionism has been a trait for me my whole life, and was a positive and a negative in my career.

It was at this point, I started to seek help through medical practitioners and psychologists. I would turn up to the doctors and burst into tears. I had an amazing doctor who helped me navigate my life at this time.

On reflection, this was a turning point for me. I was seeking help, and not just blaming myself or internalising my anxieties.

# Chapter Five: Rebuilding My Life

## Rebuilding My Life

In 2012 I took a long-term approach to rebuilding my life.

I had been experiencing Depression and Anxiety for many years. I wanted to live in Brisbane, renting a unit and get back to community work.

It started with the concept of investing. I had paid off my debts caused by youth and impulsiveness and wanted to have some independent income. One day in my kitchen, I wondered if I could apply the investment concept to my mental health recovery. Could I do something now, that might pay off in the future?

I had already been focused on practicing soft skills and characteristics. A long-term approach fitted in with this nicely.

## Long-Term Approach

I had to give up hoping for or expecting fast results. I had to give up thinking I was 'transformed for life'.

These were replaced by thoughts along the lines of:
If I can't finish something, at least make progress. Little steps add up over time.
Acknowledge that I do know my own limits. It doesn't benefit anyone to be worn out and useless for the rest of the day. Do what is comfortable, or I can do, not what I should do. Focus on realistic small steps.

To experience a sense of self, I had to look at physical things and achievements I'd made. I had a feature wall with memories and achievements on them. I'm sure my neighbours thought I was up myself. The truth was, I felt really disconnected to who I knew I could be. I felt really disconnected to who I once was. I needed something physical to say 'yes it's true. You did do those things!'

Over time I identified small goals on the path to working. My goals and to do lists were regularly updated to allow for an understanding of my limits and talents.

## Detail Oriented

Over my recovery journey, I found that I need lists of tasks. My memory for things to do can be shockingly short. I could turn around or take a few steps and I've forgotten what I've just committed to. That I even made a commitment.

At first, my lists had to be ridiculously detailed. I recall one having about twenty items on it. I would tick off which tasks I did each day.
Slowly that started to overwhelm me. I found I could put things into contexts. For instance, on my morning schedule, I now have 'Shower, dress, brush teeth & hair, take medicine, eat something small'. In the past that would have to be micro scheduled into 'Get clean clothes, put a towel in bathroom, shower, shave face, put dirty clothes away, brush teeth, dry hair, brush hair'.

Being detail oriented has helped with the various plans I've made. I've written business plans, project plans, grant applications and financial plans. Being articulate has helped with the planning processes.

I had a sign in my kitchen for a year saying 'Focus on one thing.' This remains an outlook that I use. Having Asperger's, I can easily get bogged down in details. While this is great for project planning, it's not so good when I have a big task that needs to be done.

## Accepting my Diagnosis

Talking to my sister Kat on the phone one day, she suggested that a friend thought I might have Asperger's. I researched it a bit on the Internet. It really didn't seem applicable to me. However, I filed 'Asperger's away for looking at later.

In 2013 I saw a documentary, Kids with Cameras (2004) about boys with Asperger's making stop-motion animated films. I felt I could relate to a few things, but not much.
Later in the year, I was looking through a list of interviews by Richard Fidler. One caught my eye. Always into learning something new, I started listening. By the first fifteen minutes, I strongly suspected I was on the Autism Spectrum. By the end of the interview, I knew. I am an Aspie.
The interview is with Dr. Tony Attwood. It was broadcast on 2nd February 2012. On the ABC radio information page, it is titled 'Dr. Tony Attwood turns his focus to women and girls with Asperger's'.

Who knew that females present different characteristics than males? A lot of it almost didn't match things I'd researched a couple of years ago. That was because the information was based on male characteristics. It was also clinical information when I needed actual examples of how Asperger's traits look in everyday life. If you have done your research, you will see female characteristics of Autism scattered all through this writing.

I must have listened to that interview ten times over the next year.

## Assessment

I recommend Tania Marshall's blog post on Assessing Autism Spectrum.
She has posted a useful article on how she assesses and diagnoses women on the Spectrum. If you are preparing for an assessment, this article lists things to bring to appointments.

I still (in 2017) haven't had a psychiatrist diagnosed me. I need this diagnosis to access certain supports from Disability Queensland. In some other states of Australia, a clinical psychologist is accepted for support requirements. A clinical psychologist has diagnosed me, but that is not enough. I regret that I don't have any paperwork from those sessions with him. I could bring it along to appointments with a psychiatrist.

I moved back to Brisbane in 2014. In 2016 I saw a psychiatrist for over six months. I don't think he read the referral my GP sent, or if he did, he didn't refer to it before any sessions. Having a communication disorder, I felt held back from asking for assessment questions at appointments. I did tell him three times during appointments, that I need a diagnosis.
At our last appointment, he asked what a diagnosis would look like. I was shocked and laughed in disbelief. 'Something written down' I said. I no longer see him, as I'm sick of seeing someone specifically for an assessment, and not getting one.

## Learning Social Skills

I've researched 'Females with Asperger's a lot. Or as Donald Trump would say 'I've got all the great research'. Reading the book 'Asperger's and Girls', I learned quite a few things about communication at work.

Just knowing that there were things called 'unwritten rules' and 'social skills' allowed me to begin learning these skills. I could identify patterns to people's behaviour and conversations.

## Hierarchies

I learned about hierarchies. I could see how that translated to the workplace and at school.

I didn't understand before why I could not report to the general manager at an office.

I would usually side-step the Office Manager. This was because, in a sense, I already had a relationship with the general manager. I felt this as they were usually the person who interviewed and hired me. This is where ridged thinking patterns and inability to form relationships comes in. Change of a new work relationship took a long time to get used to.

In the workplace, I had to learn that people occasionally fight and don't speak. That this did not mean the friendship was over for good. I also learned that just because someone has talked to someone else, it doesn't mean they are friends.

## Hidden Meanings

Then there was the concept of hidden meanings, and how that correlated into putting something in context. Previously I'd thought that hidden meanings were a theoretical saying. If they did exist, I'd banded them into the same group as ever-unforgivable assumptions. My years of attending personal development seminars had reinforced that you should avoid acting on assumptions. That they were like brain farts (my words).

## Being Articulate with a Social Disorder

I knew I was articulate. Hadn't enough people told me that? I had done seminars on communication with the personal development company aforementioned. I thought I had extra skills that other people didn't have. In some ways, I still think I do.

What I couldn't understand, the few times people mentioned the possibility, was that I could also have a communication disorder.

Think about making an apple pie from scratch. You could have delicious apples, by which I mean, you are articulate and choose your words carefully. However, you don't know the recipe for making the dough. Read that as, you don't know the existence of social rules, hidden meanings, hierarchies and conversational patterns. If this is you, you're going to make a rough, likely inedible apple pie.

Translated as people think you're rude, overstepping bounds on purpose, assuming intimacy that isn't there, and think you're full of yourself. The apples in and of themselves are yummy.

You are articulate still. Unfortunately, the mix and method are faulty. You are missing information.

## Being Overwhelmed

I had to learn that what I'm capable of and what I can do when overwhelmed, are sometimes polar opposites.
That if it takes 20 minutes to create an invoice in a template, I need to take a break. I am overwhelmed or exhausted and need to recover my processing abilities.
For instance, half an hour of communicating requires about an hour to recover from the intense concentration used. One hour of talking can require up to three hours of recovery. Shorter, more effective recovery comes from being in a dimly lit room, with muted sound and very little activity around me. Even if I am overwhelmed but working in silence, that will keep me overwhelmed and create more confusion.

## Recovery Star Progress

A case-worker let me know about a method of tracking your recovery progress. It is called The Recovery Star. I have been using it at various times since 2012, through to the present (2017).

The ten sections as listed below helped me identify key areas of my life to work on. It also allowed me the space to record when and where I was doing well. I'll take you through the ten sections, in no particular timeline.

**Managing Mental Health**

To be clear, I am talking about managing my Anxiety and Depression. I consider being on the Autism Spectrum as simply having another type of operating system. Neurotypical people may run Windows, while I run Mac or Linux.

Through the years I've practiced being present, mindfulness and breathing techniques.

I made having a regular Doctor (General Practitioner) mandatory. I took on counseling with psychologists.

I got various degrees of seriousness about managing my mental health through the documentaries 'Don't Call Me Crazy (The UK, 2003) and Changing Minds (AUS, 2016). I had to find out how important it is to take my medicine daily, on time. I realised that I may need them for the rest of my life.

In 2016 I wrote my own detailed mental health plan. If you are interested in this process, I blogged about writing my plan at Musings of KarlettaA.com. It can be found in the Mental Health category.

**Physical Health and Self-Care**

I am still a lot bigger than I would like but am doing what I can to be healthier.

When I'd randomly have energy, I took on walking around my backyard. I have had an app for counting my steps for about three years now. I've been doing an average of 7,000 steps per day for about a year now.

I learned how many calories I should have a maximum of per day. The main thing I did with this info is stopped buying pizzas, regular takeout and starting to drink Coke Zero or Pepsi Max instead of the full sugar versions.

I started doing exercises while in bed that are low impact. I took up working on my flexibility as I did when I did gymnastics.

## Living Skills

I learned how important visual reminders of my daily schedule are. I found out how bad my memory can be.

I learned how to make realistic, fairly easy and comfortable goals. Ableist concepts like 'you need to step out of your comfort zone to make progress' don't help my peace of mind. My body feels distressed enough most days without making myself uncomfortable on purpose.

I still have problems with organisation, executive function, being overwhelmed by household chores and self-care tasks. Thankfully I am not laid out for months though.

## Social Networks

I've been learning about many social and conversational concepts. I've learned that there are expected listening skills other than listening only to words.

Previously I had thought that body language is used to emphasize words.

I didn't know before that people use body language instead of their words. That it can be the opposite of what they say verbally.

I don't look for body language often, still finding this distressing, but can look for it occasionally.

I had to learn that there are hidden meanings in conversations. I'm pretty sure most of these are still hidden from me!
Hidden meanings I've learned include who I'm "allowed" to talk to and in which conversational style. I am not supposed to talk to a boss as I would to my friends. This still baffles me. I learned how entrenched people are about divisions between social classes, the concept of climbing the social ladder, and what the queen bee in a group does.

I may write about social skills I've discovered in a future book.

*DSM 5 Diagnostic Criteria A.2.*

*Deficits in nonverbal communicative behaviors used for social interaction, ranging, for example, from poorly integrated verbal and nonverbal communication; to abnormalities in eye contact and body language or deficits in understanding and use of gestures; to a total lack of facial expressions and nonverbal communication.*

## Work

Allowing myself to randomly write, sew, make art and craft projects, and cook labor intensive meals has been keeping me busy and give me a sense of accomplishment. I've completed about six short courses through an online website called Open 2 Study.

I've offered to volunteer at a few organisations. I did a few volunteer shifts. At times during cycles of feeling good and being productive, I've been sending off my resume for job applications. I've had no interview offers for years, however.

## Relationships

I've developed a good working relationship with my sister, who I share a house with. It has been fantastic hanging out with her and her children Annerley and Parker.

I've reconnected with my mum. For a few years, I thought she was a narcissist and lacked empathy. I've discovered recently that she actually has Asperger's. I wrote about the process of discovering this in my blog post 'Even I Misinterpreted Autistic Traits'.

I have slowly and steadily built up friendships with people in my areas of interests. They are mainly around science, writing, and females on the Autism Spectrum. I interact with my friends from years ago, though not as often as I'd like. I still find myself being unreliable with my friends.

## Addictive Behaviour

I have stopped smoking pot, but am still smoking cigarettes. Currently, I'm drinking a six pack or two a week, which is a lot less than I used to.

I have been making great strides with managing my impulsive behaviours in many areas of my life.

## Responsibilities

### My pet cat

I consider my cat as my support animal. According to my values, I've paid to get my cat microchipped, neutered, and vaccinated. I've also joined a pet care program through Green Cross Vets. For $30 a month, I can get some free and discounted vet appointments, as well as discounts for operations and many pet cares purchases. Gosh, that sounds like an advert doesn't it?

## Finances

I've paid off my debts and save money regularly. When I get too impulsive and spend it, I start saving again.

## Being a Responsible Auntie

This includes not drinking as much as I used to and doing chores with my niece and nephew.

## Identity and Self-Esteem

This one is tricky as I have an elusive sense of self. While I don't have a sense of self during chit-chat conversations, it is much easier to hold onto ideas of who I am at other times.

Specifically, when there is a purpose to the conversation or I know my role within a group activity.

Through writing about it over the years, I have developed realistic, healthy ways of thinking about my achievements and future. I don't think I can change societies anymore. It would be nice, but doubtful.

My next memoir, called Elusive Identity, is about trying to maintain a sense of self and rebuilding my identity from scratch.

## Trust and Hope

Hope is something I've had to create over and over again. I've come to recognise the differences of a goal being a hope versus a goal being an expectation. I find that expectations don't allow space to be willing to fail, learning much from the past and being as flexible as I'd like.

I am finding it easier to trust in my abilities to finish projects. Through writing these eBooks, blogging, photos of things I've achieved, and having a bit of money set aside, having physical accomplishments has helped me through feelings that I'm useless.

# Rebuilding My Life Contributions

## Kathy

I have now accepted that I need to keep working as a casual nurse in my old workplace while I develop new directions. I am building up a business.

The decision not to chase a new permanent job in my old field, with only an indifferent manager as a referee has been freeing. I still haven't told them at work; only a very few colleagues who were aware I was seeking a diagnosis. It doesn't feel like a safe place to be neurodivergent in.

I have had some counselling – that wasn't a completely unmitigated disaster, though it came close. I learned techniques for mindfulness meditation, and I also learned that psychologists don't want you to disagree with them when they make an assumption about you.

I have started exploring the idea of research in a more formal way, through doctoral study, and as a peer researcher, and am in the process of starting a business supporting autistic people to access health care services.

I had never considered the idea of running my own business before; the distress and helplessness I felt when realising my ability to gain work had been severely compromised have started opening doors I hadn't realised were there.

I know I have the ability to throw myself into something once I feel the commitment biting, and my strengths in research, in supporting people in a way that puts them at the center of their life, and my love of presenting and discussing with others who share interests with me are strengths drawn in part from my Autism.

I know there are others who have had the experience of being broken and powerless, of recognising the pattern in a lifetime of difficulty, and the struggle to rebuild lost confidence and new pathways.

## Laina

What I've done during my second and third burnouts is to become more selective when accepting patients into the practice.

I've tightened up my policies and procedures, and I've spelled them out more thoroughly. I've learned to look for "red flags" that might indicate that someone is going to be a problem. (For example, irrational, litigious, attention-seeking, combative, abusive, or manipulative people, those with unrealistic expectations, etc.).

Unfortunately, this was a very necessary step, as I've come across a lot of unreasonable people, or people who are "married to their disease" where, when the rubber meets the road, they actually don't want to get better. They might think they do, but they resist the very sound answers and plans of action I've presented to them. I have to screen people very carefully. I always make sure that there is no confusion or misunderstanding of what this approach is all about.

I want everything to be out in the open, all of us on the same page and any partners to be on board and supportive. (I don't want them to be caught in the middle between what they and I want to do, and an unsporting partner who doesn't think the patient's issues are that bad.).
I want to do right by everyone I serve and I want to feel good at the end of the day, knowing I did my very best to help people. The policies I created are extremely fair and logical. I give where I can, but I don't sell myself short anymore. When teetering in a situation, I err on the side of the patient. I've tried to be as cut and dry, but also bendable if necessary, at the same time. It's quite a tightrope to walk

I've chosen to remain low volume, and to pack my schedule into a few days per week, all in the morning when I'm at my best for meeting with people. Once I'm in "people mode", I can stay there and see another patient. But I can't deal as well with spaces in my schedule (I.e., one person at 10 am and then not another one until noon, etc.). I know that although I met with 5 people today (which is huge for me), I was finished by lunch.

I take the afternoons to interpret lab test results and research information. Or create educational handouts for patients. I'm always doing something for patients, although I only get paid for a small part of it. But I still love it.

## Liz

Once I started to seek help through the right channels, that is, doctors and psychologists, things got worse, but at the same time, better.

I was getting somewhere, and it was painful but at the same time, I needed answers. Seeking help with professionals is what set me on the road to discovering my wonderful autistic self. I would say that autism is my "special interest". I love reading everything about it and being a part of the autism advocacy and research communities. I have 2 post graduate degrees specializing in Autism, and I am pursuing future career directions in autistic research.

I miss music so much, and I have actually released some music in a different genre once my son was born. I would love to write music again, and maybe one day it will happen. But I don't miss touring, I miss traveling though. I don't miss the political games that are played in the music industry, the hidden agendas of people who say they're your friends but aren't. I don't miss self-medicating.

I am definitely a work in progress, and career-wise I am not sure where I am heading, or if I will ever venture into the music world again. Only time will tell. It will involve a lot of reflection and a lot of healing.

# Chapter Six: Where Are We Now?

## A Work in Progress

I think it's important to share my story even though my goals are incomplete.

A 2013 Australian survey by Autism Spectrum Australia found that just 54 percent of adults with Asperger's or high-functioning autism had a paid job. It also found that a third of those who are employed want more support in the workplace.

I am feeling a lot more settled, confident and sometimes even sexy. Through looking after my nutrition, medication and walking, I'm able to keep a fairly stable mood. It makes being overwhelmed and meltdowns less intense.

I am still on the disability pension. I have always regarded volunteering as working. Hence, while writing non-fiction a few days a week, I'll tell my cat 'mummy's working now. I need the chair'. My cat is my support animal and companion. He can get a bit short though when I want to sit in 'his' chair.

I'm feeling OK or good most days. There are days or weeks when I'm not well enough to manage my chores. My room can be messy more often than not. At the moment I've stopped cooking every night for my household. I feel like I'm juggling too many things.

*DSM 5 Diagnostic Criteria D.*

*Symptoms cause clinically significant impairment in social, occupational, or other important areas of current functioning.*

At times of being overwhelmed, I might go mute, retreat into my room or just silently listen to music all day. I am only concerned when I am mute for more than 24 hours. Then I know I need to see a professional or have a frank conversation with someone.

## Being Uncomfortable

I think I felt uncomfortable a lot in the past due to my communication disorder. Not only was I afraid of being socially humiliated, but I just never knew what to say. I still feel uncomfortable more than I'd like, but it's not got such a hold on me anymore.

At times I feel like a visitor to another culture. People are laughing and joking about something, but I have no idea what is going on.

Feeling uncomfortable also comes from body sensations from sensory feedback. I can feel an unpleasant tingle when I go to pick up a menu in a cafe I've never been to. I can develop an almost-headache from the brightness of a light. I can experience a sense of shock when someone suddenly, unexpectedly laughs loudly, exclaims or makes a loud sound.

## Time Management

Back when I was working on my magazine or other projects, I needed to manage my energy and take frequent breaks. I was afraid that if I stopped for too long, I would forget ideas or what I needed to do. Almost like money walking out the door!

I have honed my skills now of writing project plans and mapping out ideas. With blog posts, I write contexts, bullet points, a theme and sometimes a practical example.
I've always moved easily from one part of a project plan to another. With using Scrivener for my writing, it allows me to do this easily. It has a visual menu of chapters and sections. You can drag and drop writing if you like. It's fantastic.

Through time management I've learned the Pomerado method of timekeeping and working. The 30-minute work allotments (and breaks!) help conserve my energy and concentration.

## Impulsiveness

Working short but regular hours over time has given me confidence in my ability to finish a project. I used to be so eager to get a finished project out there. Instead, I've found value in still using those ideas, but developing them over time.

Through blogging, I've learned how to put a cap on my impulsiveness of publishing something straight away. I've discovered the joy of mapping out possible blog posts and keeping drafts unpublished. Well, joy is a bit strong. It's more like trust that posts can wait, and be again edited later.

## ADD

When I see a new psychiatrist, I will be seeking an assessment to find out if I have Attention Deficit Disorder, and if so, which type. There is a constant battle with trying to make myself hold onto the reasons for why self-care and home chores need to be done. One of my favourite Ways of Being is Being Intentional. In those times I am able to focus. Seeing as I find it incredibly hard to focus on most things, I think that I have ADHD.

When I go to do tasks like chores and self-care, I can initially know why I am doing something. I am aware of the purpose and what my end goal will be. Pretty quickly that understanding and need to complete a task dissipates. I am left stranded doing physical tasks with no feelings of why and only vague logical thoughts that the task needs to be done. The logical thoughts are not 'It makes sense to finish the dishes because then the kitchen will look clean'. The thoughts are more like 'I've promised myself to do the dishes, so I'm supposed to do them. I don't know why this is so important, but people say it is'. It is like being told that 34 x 73 is 1833, but have no logic to work this out for myself. I am told that that is the answer so I shrug and say 'If you say so. I can't see it'.

It is counter-intuitive, but at times I have to allow myself to forget the existence of such things as food, medicine and writing to be able to do self-care tasks. You may have heard the saying 'Having Asperger's is like having 100 Internet browser tabs open all the time.' All I can say is Yes, Yes, it is.

## Options for the Future

When I'm finished writing these three books, I hope to volunteer a couple of days a week and do more short courses online. In the past few years, since moving back to Brisbane, I've finished about six online courses through Open 2 Study.

Eventually, I want to return to part-time work. I would like it to be at a small office, possibly with someone that I know already. From writing my three books, I know I can work for a few hours two to three days a week.

I am still interested in studying and working in the community services sector. For example, I would love to be a Peer Support Worker. Peer support workers do individual case management with people who experience similar challenges. They have lived experiences of something. For me, it would be Depression, Anxiety, and the Autism Spectrum.

In the meantime, my writing projects and watching science videos and articles has kept me occupied and been mentally stimulating. I have made a few acquaintances in various scientific fields, which I am glad of. I'm now a member of the Queensland Museum and am looking forward to attending some of their guest evenings and exhibitions.

## Employers

Why don't I have a job now? To be frank, I don't think an employer would give a crap about my needs.

Do you remember early on how I said I had conflicting behaviours at work? I could be productive and successful for short stretches of a time and couldn't understand why suddenly I'd be worn out and unmotivated. Working and conversing requires massive amounts of concentration. It is like I am doing logic puzzles all day. I need frequent and long breaks. I may need to leave work early or take a day off here and there due to depressive states.

In an interview, I am scared to ask for frequent and long breaks during my workday. These would be mandatory. They have always been part of my workday, albeit a process I often felt guilty about. When updating my timesheets at the end of the day, I would feel guilty for recording fewer hours than I was hired for. I also can't work for more than two or three days in a row.

Traveling by bus, as I do, can be a problem. While I live in Mount Gravatt, my nearest bus only comes by once an hour. In the likely event when I'm being unreliable (read as unable to make myself do tasks), missing my bus would change my work hours. Being unmovable about certain things, I would insist on sticking to my routine and finishing work at the usual time.

I'm sure no employer would forgive these actions I've described. They would probably come back at me with ableism comments like 'We leave our troubles at home when we walk in the door.' I feel like asking for these things is demanding unrealistic things. I can clearly see and have experienced, employers who pretend to agree to my needs, but underestimate or ignore them once I'm in the office.
What I would need in those cases is a job search consultant to stand up for me, and demand these things on my behalf, over time. My experience with job network agencies has been that they don't stand up for my needs in this way.

For people who can't identify and articulate what they need? It's a massive challenge to work.

## Public Speaking

I would like to start doing short sessions of public speaking again. I would like to do these lightning talks at an Autism conference, a community information day or other places.

I've written out a speech called 'Why is that lady so nervous?' I've made notes about talks on Autistic burnout, self-identity and Gender Dysphoria, Autism and homelessness, and short-lived relationships with guys.

I've researched about building up a public speaking career, and information on booking a short spot. Now I've just got to bite the bullet and network!


## Writing Projects

I have just had a short story published in an anthology of fan fiction. It is in The Demons of Butte Crack County by author John Birmingham. I was stoked to be placed in the first half of the book.

For the past three months, I have been writing fairly consistently. My blog posts are coming out fortnightly. I have been working on three eBooks, one of which you are reading now.

At the time of this being revised and printed, I have two poetry collections, a guide to event management, and a memoir out now on Kindle. My second memoir, called "Elusive Identity" is being written.

I feel like I am part of a community of emerging writers. We can be a determined, resourceful and independent lot. Learning and a love of learning is a key part of my days.

I like being a writer.

# Where Are They Now? Contributions

## Kathy

Although I'm still working as a community palliative care nurse when the work is available, the time I spent defining myself by that has passed.
The idea of my business is still brand new (supporting autistic people to access health care services). There is a lot to do in preparation, but the juggling and the list-making are no longer overwhelming.

The reduction of depression and anxiety levels has allowed me a measure of calm and clear thought. For a few years now, I hadn't been making lists of tasks, but I now have one on the wall to remind me of the tasks yet to do when I sit down at my computer.

I work daily to keep anxiety and depression at bay. I engage in my interests; I walk with my husband – precious time alone together – I listen to my kids talk about their passions and school day. Acknowledging the issue, bringing my autism, my depression and my anxiety with me on the journey reduces the tension I felt when I was fighting and denying it.

I have my family, I have my online "tribe", and I have my passions. I have some alone time every day, and I have time to work on business ideas.

The idea of working directly with clients, and avoiding the necessity to rely on someone else's opinion of me to be able to work, is appealing and freeing. There are development opportunities for this business, and for myself, and I expect to work hard – as I always have on things I deem important.

I am on a steep learning curve with setting up a business and changing the way I do things, but I have always loved a steep learning curve, and I have supportive people around me.
I feel hopeful again, for the first time in more than two years.

## Laina

Seven years in, we're still living week to week, and month to month. We're getting by, because my 15-year-old truck is paid off and we live in a safer-but-still-reasonable apartment, and we bring our lunch from home to the office. We make sandwiches at lunchtime. We don't buy much.

I have since bounced back somewhat in the years since finishing med school, but I'm not done yet. I've since developed PTSD, realized that I have Ehlers-Danlos Syndrome (EDS) and realized that I'm an Aspie. Along with hearing loss and hemochromatosis, I also probably have Hashimoto's Disease. I'm very fortunate; I should be tired, in pain, and in a wheelchair, taking lots of meds, on disability.
But I'm not. I co-own an integrative medical practice with my partner, although it is slow-going. My Asperger's is the biggest factor in the delay except that it also makes me good at what I do.

I've learned to segregate my time. I have my "people mode", my "independent work mode", and my downtime modes, which include blogging, hanging out with the cats and my partner, talking with my parents and 2 best offline friends on the phone, checking social media, etc.

I've also learned to take short breaks throughout the day at work, to let my brain rest and recharge. These usually occur during transition times, when switching "modes". Long before I realized I was an Aspie, I started noticing the definite need for this, and I started obliging.

Now that I know I'm an Aspie, these needs (everything I've described) make total sense to me. Our business is coming along slowly but surely.

## Liz

Personally, I am on a journey of self-discovery, reflection and self-forgiveness. I work to be kinder to myself, understand myself, and give myself a break.

Professionally I am in transition. I'm not sure where I'm heading or what lies ahead, but I know now, there is more hope than before.

I am starting my doctorate this year, and it will be about autistic female entrepreneurs in creative industries, reflecting on my own experiences, discovering other experiences in this field and hopefully finding ways to help autistic females discover their own career passions in the future.

I am hoping to be an example for my son, and be an example on how to discover your strengths, and deal with your needs, without feeling bad or self-blaming. I try to seek help when I need it.

My journey is starting, my reflection is endless, and my hope is growing every day.

# About the Authors

# Notes from the Author

Thank you for reading my book. I hope you saw a bit of yourself in our stories. That you feel known and valuable. I would love to hear back from you!

Please review it. It helps others find it. Please leave a review of at least 10 words, as I find short ones unhelpful when shopping.

You can follow my writing and provide feedback on future manuscripts by subscribing to my email list at http://eepurl.com/cBDCmH

I try to blog fortnightly at www.MusingsofKarlettaA.com

# Blog posts

# Masking and powering on when I didn't realise, I am Autistic #Takethemaskoff

I have this picture, or used to have, of me just before a short speech at a launch of a youth service.

A piece of paper is in front of me, on a desk, and I am looking up to the camera. I am in the middle of writing a speech.

I am in a red tee-shirt with short sleeves, a broad grey stripe across my chest. My chest is relatively flat because I bound my breasts. I am wearing blue jeans and black boots. A bright red cap is on my head, with an unimportant logo on it.

I remember the day vividly. It is one of the first times, if not the first time, that I drafted a speech. Usually, I'd just wing it, getting on stage and assuming I would know what to say.

This time however, I want to be more professional. I'm only feeling slightly nervous as I revise and rewrite the speech.

I am in my own little world, the only accompaniment are people in my imagination, responding to things I may say – a clap here, a handshake after, and finally telling people what I want them to know about me. I'm trying to get ready for any eventuality. I don't want to be looked at with scorn today. This is a big day.

Finally, I finish. I relax then gaze around the room, slowly.

There are quite a few people attending this launch. Maybe forty or fifty. A number of them are gathered around a long table with food on it. 'Food', the thought is clear and gives me a direction.

Only then do I realise that I am hungry. I either couldn't afford too much food at the time, given my uneven spending habits, or I just didn't want to waste time eating when I could be preparing for today.

I look at the plates on the table, one by one, noticing the different types of sandwiches, the various rolls of sushi, and taking my time deciding what drink I feel like. I load my plate, spend a minute eating in my own little world.

Then start noticing things people are saying. I hear their voices, each pitched differently, some slower, some faster, some excited, some people sound bored.

The people surrounding me and the sounds from every direction is disorienting. I listen until something sounds familiar. A lady's voice reaches through the mess and I find it easy to grasp. I inch my way over, looking at her occasionally. Aah, she's talking about youth homelessness. I know about this; I live in temporary accommodation after all. I almost had to live on the streets one night.

I speak as confidently as I can, masking that I have no idea how to start a conversation with this woman. With this group. I speak, probably too loudly, letting her know I understand what she means. Looking surprised, she smiles, and asks me who I am. I hand over my business card 'I run a magazine' I say. 'It's called Cookies'.

Now I don't know what to say. A handful of things swirl in my head, competing for my attention. They all sound trite, or possible things to be ridiculed for.

I try my best to not show fear on my face, just smile knowingly at the group conversation. This stranger might laugh at me when this event is over. I've got to be nice and make a good impression.

When the confusion gets too much, when I can't think of anything to say other than a jumble of words, I say my goodbyes, thanking her for her time, and hoping she will call me about a public speaking gig.

My heart races, I am disoriented, and look around for someone familiar. Someone who I can connect a feeling to. I find someone. I introduce myself to someone I don't know in the group. I ask a question, and I listen, able to follow the group's sentences, but unable to figure out what to contribute. The lady I know, her familiar voice, the way she structures her sentences, her values are familiar and soothing. My muscles slowly untighten, my heart beat feels softer, and I calm down again.

Ooh, the event is starting 'Soo soon?' I think. I've just started meeting people! Well, here we go.

The youth service is described, the need for it is palpable for me. I feel like this group of people have one mind. We want to make a safe space for young Lesbian, Gay, Bisexual, Transgender and Intersex people (LGBTI). Kids are getting bullied at school, their parents angrily dismiss them, they have limited space to relax and just speak their minds. At the event, we know that, or we should. I wonder who here doesn't have much experience with hanging around LGBTI young people? People from Department of Housing maybe? Other youth service workers? Who knows? There's got to be a few here.

It's my turn to speak. My nerves build up as I walk to the stage, up the stairs. The moment I step onto the stage, I relax. I am in front of people, knowing their attention is on me, uninterrupted. These people are interested in what I have to say.

Well, I have plenty to say. I look at my notes – what to say first, what comes next, how to end it. I introduce myself and there is clapping. My body betrays me and my cheeks tighten and move up into a grin. I am blushing and broadly smiling in wonder. 'Stop it!' I think. 'You're here to talk'. So, I talk. I share how I am transgender – a female to male. I have been homeless, and this house I'm in is my third supported housing service I've needed. This service has already helped me feel less alone. Given me somewhere safe to hang out.

Back then, I probably looked at people as a group. Not focusing in on any one person, with one exception. He is on the board of the housing service where I am living. At one point I mention them 'Prospect House' and look at him, so he knows that he is being acknowledged. I don't know what I talked about that day. I just know that there was laughter once. I finished my speech, stepped down to applause, and stood next to the board member. I felt we had shared a moment of acknowledgement. He saw me on stage, and I saw him helping LGBTI youth.

Afterwards, I made my way to the food table, and introduced myself to a few more people. 'Did you hear me? I can do speeches for you guys you know. Here's my card' was the general drift.

After a while, utterly exhausted, I leave and sit at the Fortitude Valley train station for a while. I just need some peace and quiet.

I did a speech recently in June 2018.

I'd prepared by brainstorming, outlining, and recording audio drafts. I listened to the final draft a few times. On the day, I fidgeted way more than I'd like. I am still very proud.

I didn't force myself to talk to strangers. I knew what Masking was this time. Knew the Anxiety, Depression, and burnout it has caused me. I left when the room of about 15 people felt crowded and suffocating.

I slept for the rest of the day.

I was aware of my limits and to let my overactive mind time to settle down. I was not hounded by shame that I was exhausted afterwards.

Just allowed myself space to recover, in peace.

# My VERY MIS-guided "understandings" about Autism and Asperger's

When I was diagnosed as Autistic in about 2012, my reaction was anger and disgust "I'm not a f****** retard".

I think I snorted when the Clinical Psychologist asked if I wanted to talk about it.

For the next two years I had no understanding of why he came to that assessment conclusion.

What do you know about Classic Autism, Asperger's, and Autistic Savants? It turns out I was incredibly mistaken and ill-informed.

*I am articulate and I have a communication disorder. You can hear my stuttering, multiple false starts, and long pauses in this interview on the Yenn Purkis Autism Show.*

*https://www.podbean.com/media/share/pb-mr7i8-ab0dff*

I am intelligent, love learning, have an advanced vocabulary, am detail-oriented, creative, caring and compassionate, and enjoy quite a few passions.

I am nothing like what I thought Aspies were. Yet I am Autistic.

These were my very misguided "understandings/ truths/ beliefs" about Autism, Asperger's, and Autistic Savants.

## Autism/ Classic Autism

You are trapped in your mind and couldn't communicate verbally or have extremely limited verbal skills.

We had to be wheelchair bound with limited and jerky movements.

Possibly could communicate with a device, and may need a helping hand to use one.

Can go to school but god knows what we do with that information.

In this case one "obviously looked" Autistic.

## Asperger's

Asperger's, I thought, was once again "blatantly obvious".

We couldn't ever make or hold eye contact.

Every single thing we said was inappropriate.

We are very slow or resistant to learning social skills.

A limited range verbally, or noticeably low intelligence, or very slow talkers.

Can have echolalia (repeating words or sentences).

Possibly can be employed or volunteer, and extra special care needs to be given so we don't get overwhelmed and throw a hissy fit or get aggressive.

Often desperate to make friends, but doesn't care about their feelings.

## Autistic Savant

Either a child (a boy or occasionally a girl) or a male professor/ scientist.

A savant was someone who said and did embarrassing things at work, home, and with their few friends.

Possibly noticeably eccentric and with zero or very limited interest in making friends.

They are extremely intelligent and organised in some areas – at work/ their passion/ gifts – but very disorganised at home. They needed a carer or a very supportive wife to look after them at home.

## Who I Am?

Autistic/ Asperger's/ an Aspie/ on the Spectrum

Sometimes have Asperger's-noticed-traits to others.

I have a few special interests. I love learning in detail about a wide range of subjects. Encyclopedias are now replaced by Wikipedia, Google, and YouTube.

As a child, I stopped speaking between the ages of four to six years old.

When overwhelmed it is possible to suspect that I am Autistic, "shy", "a bit nervous ", or "just stutters sometimes".

Please, for the love of cute kittens, remove the term "High-Functioning Autism" from your vocabulary. I identify as low to medium functioning. Or, you know, Karletta.

My Autistic traits are ignored by or hidden from observers – not myself (anymore) – for self-preservation.

## Inexplicably Shy

I consider myself as outgoing, a networker, and a public speaker. It didn't make sense to me why I would "turn shy ". Now, I know.

Humiliation or the threat of being seen as "pathetic", "over reacting" or "too much work" for others has me acting "shy".

## I need to recharge often

I have been taught in millions of heartbreaking lessons to be ashamed of and hide my "pathetic" characteristics and sensitivities.

Crowds, loudness, brightness affect me physically and emotionally. At a conference recently, I learned how freeing it is to wear foam earplugs and sunglasses out in public.

I know nowadays how important breaks are for settling racing thoughts, energy restoration, memory retention, and socialising.

Closing my eyes, and/ or keep my head down while listening soothes and rests my senses. At school, when I did that, teachers would clap loudly and demand I "wake up and pay attention." All this would do is increase my anxiety, and lessen my attention and memory abilities until my next restorative rest.

The confrontation of being demanded to repeat what a teacher has just said got me defensive, and my thoughts shut down.

## Inexplicably couldn't work anymore

This masking and refusal of others to understand and happily fully support Autistic employees causes Autistic burn out and regression.

I went through it, am still experiencing its effects a decade later. I thought I was the only one, and wrote a memoir about Autistic burnout. I made sure to collect experiences from others who've been or are burnt out. (Ryan Boran has an amazing piece on his blog with many references and quotes about burnout and its long-term ramifications.)

*Autism awareness and acceptance month sounds nice. What I would love is Autism Appreciation month, as Tori Haar suggested recently.*

*https://www.westpac.com.au/news/in-depth/2019/04/changing-the-autism-conversation/*

I am intelligent, love learning, have an advanced vocabulary, am detail-oriented, creative, caring and compassionate, and enjoy quite a few passions.

I am nothing like what I thought Autism/ Aspies were.

I have worked full-time, part-time, and volunteered.

Historically I have had extreme difficulty finding and retaining a permanent home. Homeless, in fact, through couch surfing, living with family, in emergency accommodation, in supported accommodation, and stuck in unsuitable leases.

I have blossomed by being in a stable, permanent rental unit. I love living by myself.

## Social skills

I am gullible and impressionable at times. I have learned to be wary of and recognise red flags of people and information.

I can be very shy/ Stutter/ Go mute due to multiple racing thoughts vying for attention and expression. I do this while talking with friends, tired, in medical appointments and emergencies, also when I am eager to not be humiliating to others.

I have to relearn all of my social skills and learned social constructs, since doing a self-development course that has you doubt *every single thing* you know about yourself/ others/ life.

I maintain eye contact often and for significant periods. Especially when I know my role/ task/ goal in that activity/ place.

## My Skills Come and Go

All sorts of my skills come and go depending on my physical, mental, and emotional health. It also depends on a situation and whether I have a purpose or role in an activity.

I need support to manage/ organise the many areas of my life, and at times am extremely self-motivated and organised at home and at work.

Organisation and motivation for doing basic life skills is rare or comes and goes like a rollercoaster. I also suspect I have ADD (Attention Deficit Disorder).

## Determined and resilient

I really like my values, skills, and that I keep picking myself up again.

I like to experiment with many life skills.

I am nothing like what I thought Autism/ Aspies were.

Boy am I glad of the years of effort that adult Autistic advocates and bloggers have made. You helped me understand myself, far, far more than any medical professional has.

Thank you. I hope your words live on forever.

# Realistic goals: A talk on realistic goals, willingly failing and practicing

The audio for this blog post can be found at my audio blog Musings of KarlettaA

This is a talk I wrote in one of my good weeks while experiencing Autistic Burn Out. Using this method as a baseline has helped me on my recovery journey with depression and anxiety.

Parallel Workshop: "Your year in review and new goal setting"
Audience: People with Autism, Depression & Anxiety
Keywords

- Realistic to you
- Practicing and being willing to fail


Hi, how are you?

My name is Karletta Abianac, and I live in Brisbane.

I live in my own rental unit and I love being surrounded by nature and the peaceful streets.

I'm really happy to be here today, talking with you. It's been years since I've done public speaking, and I'm really glad to be back on stage again!

In my youth I used to volunteer and do public speaking about disadvantaged youth, then became a seminar leader for a personal development company.

I had to stop public speaking and working in 2006, when my depression and anxiety became too intense to manage. I wrote a memoir about the experience called Successful to Burnt Out. Successful to Burnt Out: Experiences of Women on the Autism Spectrum (I've been there too, Darl Book 1)

I have five self-published books now, and after years of practice, am happy to call myself a writer.

Talking to you, is a sign that I'm over the worst of my burn out. So, I'm really glad to be here, sharing some helpful stuff about how I've been achieving my goals.

I'm going to be talking today about how to recognise unrealistic goals, and create ones that you're comfortable with.

I asked you to come along today with a goal in mind. Or maybe you have an unwanted habit that you are trying to break?

Who here has got a goal that feels like it's a good idea and you SHOULD do it? Please raise your hands.

Who here has got a goal that feels completely achievable? Please raise your hands.

Keep your hand up if they are the same goal.

The three things I will be talking about are goals realistic to you, and being willing to fail, and practicing.

If you find yourself practicing new habits some or all of the time – on a regular basis, then give yourself a pat on the back. In fact, why don't you acknowledge and celebrate your efforts for the rest of the day. Today is your day to celebrate your efforts and your commitment.

You are not starting from scratch at this speech. You are building on the experiences of your previous goals.

You will hopefully find today really helpful for a few reasons.

One – you will see some pitfalls that we can get into – traps that take you away from practicing and achieving your goals.

The second reason is you may learn things that help you be successful this time around at practicing your goals.

Thirdly, I hope that you will feel comfortable about updating your current goals.

If you just cannot motivate yourself to change a habit or behaviour, today could be a special day for you too.

I'll talk about some reasons why we fail to achieve our goals. Chances are, you'll realise why you stopped practicing.

If you have executive function challenges, Attention deficit disorder and other health challenges – this is NOT going to radically alter your life. But it will help you recognise unrealistic goals for you.

To start off with, Expectations kill off our desire and motivation to keep practicing new habits.

I hear that we live in a world of instant gratification. I know I certainly feel this.

This includes having unrealistic expectations – for instance, if you are working on changing a habit, what may be realistic for you is to stop yourself from doing an old behaviour once or twice a week.

Or if you want to start exercising, what might be realistic for you is to just spend time stretching every few days.

One way that I started to get fitter a few years ago was to just do stretching in bed every few days. Then I moved to exercises in a chair, then walking around my veranda and doing gymnastics warm-ups. Later I started walking around my back yard.

For people who've spent years practicing giving up unwanted habits, it still often takes them months to change a habit for good.

For myself, I typically spent a week just observing myself – noticing when I was doing a bad habit.

Then I would spend a fortnight being willing to fail at stopping myself from doing that habit.

Then the next few months would be spent practicing not only stopping myself, but also replacing the bad habit regularly. Or with a goal, working on an outcome regularly.

For myself right now, I am to write for 10 minutes a day. That is far more realistic, and feels more comfortable than my old goal of writing 1,000 words a day.

We tend to think that once we commit to changing a bad habit, we should be able to stop doing it every time.

It really doesn't work that way. Letting go of a bad habit involves a lot of practice and a lot of failed attempts.

You can cut yourself some slack. You really are allowed to.


When assessing your goals and revising them, don't give up exploring and practicing ideas you have. Something that didn't work months ago might work today, because you are in a different frame of mind.

There are also things that you've learnt over the past few months that you don't realise you've learnt until you give it another go.

You cannot know whether something will work until you try it. Well, I think that's too strong a statement. Sometimes we have a pretty good idea that we can't do something. Maybe we are constantly forcing ourselves to do something. Just revise your goal – how realistic is it for you, right now?

There are a few stages to achieving a goal and changing bad habits that work for me.

## 1) Acknowledge your headspace

What are your expectations? Do you think you should stop unproductive habits in a matter of weeks? Do you think you need to achieve a goal next week? Can you take the pressure off and have it done within a few months instead?

How realistic does your goal feel to you? Not how realistic do you think it is for a person, the neighbour, the person sitting next to you. How realistic do you feel it is for you, right now, at this stage in your life?

Being someone with depression or anxiety, you could give yourself a week or two to notice and just observe yourself doing an unwanted habit. Practice mindfulness by separating yourself from your expectations.

Wouldn't that take the pressure off you to get it right all the time?

You are going to have days when you are on fire and do heaps. Just let them happen naturally, and get on with doing what you can in the meantime. Manage your expectations when you think this SHOULD be the new normal.

* Write down something that you're ok with noticing, practicing, and failing.

## 2) Support Structures

Is your environment toxic? Maybe there are people around you that you'd really rather not want to be friends with.

Is your environment aligned with your goal? Try having an ample supply of cleaning products, putting your medication in a week long pill boxes, having a favourite scented soap and shampoos.

What written structures do you have for recording your practicing, and your fails and successes? By default, we usually easily remember the failures, and feel there are more than you've had.

I've been recording some of my failures and success over the years. Some journal entries, budgets, notes, daily schedules and to do lists. I've found it invaluable to look back on them months and years later. I can see unrealistic expectations and short-term goals that should have been allotted more time.

If you've got them somewhere, bring out your old budgets and to do lists. See what you can learn from the past.

* Write down what concerns could you get rid of that free you up to practice or achieve your goal?

## 3) Practicing

Try practicing and failing, instead of expecting perfection and failing. We practice to build the mental muscles to be able to do it on command.

You don't need a big outcome in mind when you're practicing. I've found it more effective to practice just for the enjoyment and sake of practicing.

Try to take a step forward, and hope your little achievements help in the long term.

Be willing to fail. Failing is simply 'not doing what you set out to do'. Practicing assumes you will fail many times until you have mastered something.

These little achievements can be times when you practice mindfulness – paying attention to what you are doing, as you are doing it.

Once again, at this stage, sometimes you will be free to take lots of actions, and sometimes you won't be. Even after you've had a great couple of weeks, or done a task a few times in a row, sometimes we stop for a while. That's part of practicing and building your mental habit muscles.

* Write down how many weeks you can give yourself for observing yourself when you try a goal, and how many weeks you will practice your updated goal or habit.

Please take a couple of minutes to update your goals. Remember to give yourself time to practice and fail, and to be as realistic as possible.

Thank you.

# What pisses me off about Simon Baron-Cohen's Autism Assessment and Clinical Guideline Recommendations

I just saw another of the many posts in a secret women's Autism support group asking where on earth can she find a Psychiatrist that will actually assess her for Autism.

Here is my reply:

*"No idea mate. The two I saw in Brisbane in the past maybe 5 years were a) didn't read my referral, didn't bother to assess me, and his only report was a private letter to my GP (that I couldn't give to any services),*
*b) a guy in who literally said "You're not getting an assessment until you've seen a speech pathologist." and "I don't think you have Autism.""*

Here is the thing – if someone is asking for an Autism Assessment, they are:

* At the end of their rope,

* Possibly in the pits of depression or Autistic Burnout,

* Unable to cope with the responsibilities and tasks in their lives.

These initial recommendations by Simon Baron-Cohen in the document titled *"Autism spectrum disorder in adults: diagnosis and management Clinical guideline*"* are utterly simplistic AND exclusionary.

*(Published: 27 June 2012 nice.org.uk/guidance/cg142)

Info in the comprehensive assessment section should be used for EVERY SINGLE PERSON asking for an assessment.

My recommendations:

1. Skip to *NICE 1.2.8 Complex*

2. Do a comprehensive assessment including history of bullying at school, being excluded, internalised shame body language, having sex with reluctant (not enthusiastic) consent, anorexia and bulimia, Ehlers-Danos Syndrome (EDS), and every assessment idea in his document with NOTHING LEFT OUT.

3. Give the person a written (minimum three (3) page assessment) result with explanations. They will need this urgently and, in the future, to be supported.

## Resources for you

*"Dear Dr: Re-requesting support, and my communication difficulties"*

*"Dear Dr: Asking for a comprehensive Autism Assessment"*

*https://musingsofkarlettaa.com/2018/11/18/dear-dr-re-requesting-support-and-my-communication-difficulties/*

*If you need an Advocate to talk to your nurse, GP, or other health professional, I recommend Kathy from Access Health Autism.*

*http://accesshealthautism.com.au/about-us/*

# Getting used to places

*This is a post on silence, observation, and relaxing.*

The audio for this blog post can be found at my audio blog
Musings of KarlettaA

The other night I got a train home. For the first time in ages. At
night.

I was nervous. Walking across some tracks on a pedestrian
crossing, anxiety bloomed. "Normal people don't feel this" I
thought. 🌋

I kept walking onto the platform. My heart racing and pulsing. My
head feeling funny. Then uncomfortable and busy. I was in a kind
of daze.

It took a while to orient myself with what to do.

I looked around at everything on the platform. Looked at each
thing until I could feel myself using it.

My eye caught on the timetable 🪧 and I took a while reading it.
familiarising myself with it.

I saw the water station. "Water!" I thought, filling my bottle.

"I must wait now" I felt, looking for seats running down the
conductor's building.

I sat. Waited. ⏳ In silence. My head was too busy for external
output. I needed to process my racing thoughts, give them time to
fall into place.

But not so silent. I heard a truck passing by. Traffic. The pedestrian crossing. 🚦I looked at that for a while, listening. I began to notice patterns. Mechanisms. These sounds felt comforting after a while. Engineering and electronics were keeping people safe. 🚧

My attention moved on. Now I acquainted myself with the sights. The half empty lot next door. The bunches of trees around the place. 🌳 Nature. 🌳 I like nature. 🌳 Being surrounded by it. 🌳

📢 "In two minutes the Cleveland train will be approaching the station. Please stand behind the yellow safety line."

Those words. How many times I'd heard them? Hundreds? Not for many years, but they were vivid. Etched in my memories. A sense of peace came over me. ☺

Another announcement. The train gets closer as my heartbeat quickens. The train slows, as do my thoughts and pulse rate.

As the people trickled, then streamed off the platform, and through a pedestrian crossing, I saw a curious thing. People walking fast, then slowing down. "Environmental factors" I thought. "What could they be?" 🗼⚱

The departing train was going past on the other set of rails. While the train passed, people quickened while crossing the tracks. They then slowed down when it had gone, and again when reaching the sidewalks.

"So, everyone gets anxious when they're on train tracks". With that explanation I was not feeling as separate from other people. A barrier pulled down.

When a train pulls up to my side of the platform, 🚃 anxiety rises sharply again. Just considering standing up and near the train exponentially rises it some more.

"Stay" I thought. "Your seat is safe". I kept sitting until the train had almost stopped. Walking to the nearest door, I noticed the absence of imagining the train will hit me. When the train stopped, my anxiety dropped sharply. I felt peaceful again.

Being on the train felt comforting. Like I was going home in a safe place. I don't often feel like this. It was lovely.

## Get used to your surroundings

If you are scouting areas in advance or trying to get used to a place, sit in silence. Take your time to listen to the sounds, and get familiar with the sights and smells of an area.

Allow your natural interest and wonder to rise. Look for patterns. Us Aspies can be great at finding patterns.

Feeling at home came with a feeling of knowing what is going on around me and why.

## Social Stories to Familiarise

I'm glad I got there early. I got to hear sounds and see patterns that govern people's behaviour – including my own.

If you're a parent using social stories with your kids, ask yourself "Do I do this?" Do you allow your child to sit in utter silence? Wait. Listen. Watch. Really get familiar with a place?

> *When someone is going through a storm, your silent presence is more powerful than a million empty words.*
> *Thema Davis, Smile & Shine*

Don't be chatting away to them. Don't use their one sentence observations and questions become a conversation. Let them gradually get comfortable.

Let our beautiful minds work as they naturally do. Let us sit in silence.

# My Autistic Burn Out and Recovery

The audio version of this blog post from Musings of KarlettaA is on Castbox FM, Spotify, Stitcher, or hopefully your favourite podcast player...

**Prelude**

I went through burnout. In some ways I'm a much stronger person from it. In some ways I'm weaker. I have been reticent to blog about Autistic Burnout.

This is mainly because I have an eBook on a number of online stores (and free audiobook) on it and I was afraid that I couldn't come up with enough original content – that isn't in the book.

Right now, it seems silly not to, so here goes my thoughts.

**The Only One**

Until I started getting stories for my memoir from other women of their burn out experiences, I thought I was the only one who'd experienced it.

Theoretically I knew that there must be other people like me, but I'd only met one person who had to stop working when they crashed.

*There is an online study about burn out experiences.*

*"You are invited to participate in research aiming to clarify the nature of burnout, as well*

*as to develop a tool to accurately measure the condition."*

*Research by the Black Dog Institute and University of New South Wales.*

That one person who was also no longer working, was a musician that I met in Rockhampton, Queensland. I felt such a connection to him. He had also won awards. He had also published, or should I say, released original work.

By the time I met him I had written two eBooks, published a street magazine and won an award from the Queensland Government.

I dearly wanted to talk to him more at a later date, but felt deeply that I had nothing to say to him. I never knew what to say to anyone – why would he be any different?

**Feeling Trapped**

Once again, a sense of shame, isolation and feeling trapped by my thoughts ruled the day.

The years after I crashed were incredibly frustrating to me. I could vividly see myself working, chatting with friends and cleaning the house, but rarely could make myself bridge the gap from imagining to doing so.

Feelings of 'This feels wrong', 'I'm sick of forcing myself' and 'No one will care anyway' were intrusive and strong.

Often my body would rebel at attempts to move. I might get a feeling of dread wash over me, or a painful lightning network run through my brain, or a prickling sensation in my limbs. I may simply be exhausted and hated forcing my heavy limbs to obey.

## Recovery

I've written a number of posts on my long recovery process so I'll link to them here.

Nope: A turning point in my mind

My talk on realistic goals, practicing, and failing willingly

My Recovery Journey

Writing my Mental Health Plan

On Confidence and Feeling Settled

## Being Productive in 2017

I've been able to be productive this year, which has been wonderful for my sense of confidence and dignity.

Sure, I'll have stretches of doing nothing, of depressive states, but I always ask for help and do something productive in the end. Within a month anyway.

### I'm Socialising Now

Truth be told, I spend quite a bit of time at home still. I have learned to relax more with being social online. I know more of what is expected of me to do and not do. For instance, to not spam people and groups with my books and blog posts. Ask questions.

I have also been doing more community activities this year than in the past.

For two weeks I went to a drop-in centre four days a week. There I reconnected with a sense of identity at times. Sometimes it's true that you see yourself in the eyes of other people.

These past weeks I've joined Facebook writers' groups, which has been validating and a great source of information.

## It's Nice to be Me

I'm not really sure how to end this post, other than to say, it's been nice meeting people this year.

It's nice to be me.

It's nice not to be fully burnt out!

## Further Reading

The Autistic Advocate's detailed long read on Autistic burnout

An Autistic Burnout

Article by Gabriela Tavella & Gordon Parker

How to tell if you're really in burnout

Silent Wave's story

(My) Asperger's / autism and burnout (?)

Jax Blunt's blog post resource list

Autistic Burn Out, Regression, Inertia and Recovery

Ryan Boren's blog post

Autistic Burn Out: The Cost of Coping and Passing

Karletta's memoir on Autistic Burn Out

Successful to Burnt Out: Featuring experiences of autistic women

Buy on Amazon, Kobo, Barnes & Noble, and other online bookstores.

Free audiobook available on Castbox FM, Spotify, Stitcher, or hopefully your favourite podcast player.

# On Confidence and Feeling Settled

For those of you who don't know, I am working
on writing eBooks for Kindle.
They are Successful to Burnt Out: Experiences of Females on the
Autism Spectrum, Inaccessible: Poetry about things inaccessible
to me, and My Life As I See It: A Young Adult.

Two of them were mostly written in years past and just needed
revising.  One of them I wrote from scratch recently.
The draft which requires a major overhaul is my autobiography.
Splitting it into a couple of eBooks is in progress.

**Being Confident**

I've noticed that I was a lot more positive about myself in the
years that I wrote the autobiography.

I know that I was putting my best foot forward so to speak. That
was intentional. However, I also remember a difference between
the confidence I had for my future, and the cynicism I have had
for several years.

Some experiences since July have been great for bringing to my
self-identity levels of confidence. Rereading my autobiography is
another experience.

I enjoy some confidence *in my future* now. I used to hope that I
wouldn't fall into another major depressive state. Nowadays my
anxiety has mellowed out into wondering, when my mood falls,
how many days I will be unproductive, anxious and out of it.

**Being Settled**

I have been feeling more and more settled since August 2016,
when I started seeing mental health professionals again.

One expression of this is feeling at home in a community of emerging writers.

Writing for this many months has been gratifying. Mainly because I've learned not to burn myself out. Going slow and steady seems to be serving me well.

For the eBook Successful to Burnt Out, I received the first couple of contributions from a woman on the Spectrum. The time and care that she took while writing her stories was fantastic.

* Here comes shameless self praise

I wonder if, in part, she was influenced by the question prompts I sent her. There are questions for each section.

I feel settled that I've done a task beyond what was expected of me. Something that *could* come in handy.

## Feeling at Home

Thanks for reading if you made it to the end. I will take virtual high fives on Twitter. Not Facebook.

Heh, only kidding.

I'll leave you with songs that have been on my playlists recently. Thanks for listening.

## An emerging writer

Drinking in L.A. by Bran Van 3000.

## Feeling settled

Home by Edward Sharpe and the Magnetic Zeros.

# Steps on my Recovery Journey

It is 2016 as I'm writing this. I have been recovering from another bout of Depression. I have been dealing with a series of them since about 2004.

Depression was part of my crash when I experienced Autistic burn out from about 2007/2008.

Over the years of my recovery journey, I've learned not to expect big results in a few months. Instead I tried to have a long-term outlook.

*My thoughts always come back to:*

*What can I learn?*

*What can I practice?*

*How can I invest now for my future?*

This long-term outlook has paid off as I'm on a long stretch of feeling like small things I've practiced are all coming together. I've emerged from the worst of my Depression and Anxiety. Now all that's left on my goals list is to return to volunteer (or paid!) work and start dating again.

This is a big difference to trying to survive each endless, tiring day.

## Recovery Star

The reasons for my Depression are multi-layered. I have learnt to think of my life in segments. I don't know if you've heard of the Recovery Star?

*The Recovery Star developed by the Mental Health Providers Forum, is an outcomes measure which enables people using services to measure their own recovery progress, with the help of mental health workers or others.*
*Sept 10, 2009*

*Recovery Star | Mental Health Partnerships*

I've found the Recovery Star helpful in assessing where I am at and identifying areas to take action on.
I'll touch on a few practical things that I've done in my journey, other than the Star, to aid me in feeling like a worthy member of society again.

## What have I learnt?

### That I need external support

Through watching the documentaries Changing Minds (AUS) and Don't Call Me Crazy (UK) I learned how important it is to keep taking my medication daily – for life if needed.

The documentaries also showed me how important it is to regularly be in counselling – even when I feel I don't need it anymore.

I'm now seeing a psychologist regularly, who I view as my safety net. She is very experienced in working with people on the Autism Spectrum (like myself) and is also adding to my conversation skills.

## That I'm not a bad conversationalist.

I've talked with two university students recently on subjects as diverse as Logic, fame, mental health, writing and American systemic racism. They were absolutely fascinating people that I'm glad I've now connected with.

## That I want and need friendships.

I know that a good quality conversation can impact my wellbeing for days. What I came to realise is that I also want a companion. I'd like someone to talk with as I'm cooking and doing the dishes.

## That I can write my own Mental Health Plan

To quote from an up and coming post on writing my own Mental Health Plan:

> *"In March 2016 I was once again facing the*
> *frustration of having to start explaining*
> *everything again from scratch. I was also*
> *disappointed by the simplistic mental health*
> *plan my GP and I had just made.*
>
> *In researching what else could be in mine, I*
> *ended up on the Queensland Health's website*
> *and its page of guidelines for Doctors."*

I wrote my own Mental Health Plan. It has given me a safety net when I get overwhelmed in appointments."

It also ended up giving me an unexpected confidence in my writing abilities. I have applied for admin jobs for word processing documents and letter dictation.

# What have I practiced?

With practicing comes being willing to fail. For me the two go together like smoked salmon and avocado.

## Rebuilding hope

I've learned to see rebuilding my life again and again as learning curves. I try to identify the contributing factors of my relapses and practice essential life skills.

I imagine it as building on neural pathways. Trying to turn them from dirt tracks into bikeways.

## How I've been preyed on

I've learned how and why many men used and discarded me when I wanted a boyfriend.

I learned warning signs of manipulation, how misogyny is such a huge part of western cultures and about rape cultures.

Through learning these things I've been able to develop confidence to get to know more men and (shock! horror!) freedom to feel sexy.

## Various skills

I've been learning a number of skills in different disciplines.

These include writing non-fiction, Direc notations in Quantum Mechanics, audio and video file creation, drawing and business planning to name a few.

Some of them have come in handy. For the Mental Health Plan, I wrote, I used a S.W.O.T. analysis of myself as an employee. (S.W.O.T. stands for Strengths, Weaknesses, Opportunities and Threats.)

# Invest Small Steps in my Future

This concept has been handy when it's time for self-care and household responsibilities.

I've had to force myself to do things when I don't see any benefit to them – in the hope that one day my actions may pay off.

## By preparing my skills for special occasions

I started wearing make up a while ago, so when I'd eventually go to something worthy of makeup, it wouldn't look too bad.

It has been nice getting dressed up to the nines. I think it's paying off!

I tried to take on a golden rule that I heard an older lady say a few months ago. "I never go out without my jewellery and hair done."

## By practicing budgeting

I took on budgeting (when I remembered), even when I don't follow my budget.

Back in 2014 when I took this mindset on, I was budgeting infrequently, and usually not following it. The point of investing little steps at a time is for the pathway to grow stronger over time.

In 2016 I've been doing a weekly budget and mostly sticking to them.

## By dressing nicely in case, it helps

Another small way of investing in my future self is showering or dressing nicely when it makes no sense that people would judge you for not doing it.

Once again, practicing something in the off chance that they pay off. In this case in case dressing nicely changes my brain into feeling more confident. It doesn't make sense to me that people would use this to judge me on my capabilities. I would have thought potential would be seen through my past achievements, intelligence or kindness.

## Where am I now?

Dressing nicely and putting on jewellery daily.

Putting on makeup a couple of days a week.

Socialising more out of the house and on social media.

Chores are tedious but am finishing them instead of chores being endless to do and neverendingly repetitive.

Using public transport and going on activities a lot more.

Thoughts that it's possible to be dating.

Developed social circle in my areas of interest (writing, science, community work).

Have a comprehensive Mental Health Plan.

My journey to feeling this well has been long with many twists and turns. My series of depressive episodes just keep rolling in and I keep getting back up again.

I hope your journey can be as rewarding.

# On writing my own Mental Health Plan

I'm writing about the process and benefits of writing my own Mental Health Plan.

A number of people have told me to talk to my General Practitioner (GP) about getting a Mental Health Plan. I have done so a number of times, but the plans seemed basic and missing important information.

It is necessary in Australia for me to have a GP made Mental Health Plan in order to access affordable mental health care.

I've been dealing for years with being on the Autism Spectrum, along with Depression and Anxiety.

## Having simple plans was frustrating

I've been frustrated over the years by the simplistic information the various GP's have asked about and recorded.

Early this year I was going through a very tough time. I wanted to admit myself to hospital. Having no suicidal intent, I knew from past experience that those efforts would be fruitless.

## Repeating my story was frustrating

Mainly accessing the free public mental health facilities in Brisbane, I had found myself time and time again having to repeat my stories, feelings and experiences. This is because staff are regularly replaced or moved on at the mental health clinics. It wasn't helped by the fact that I was bouncing from share house to share house.

Having to explain myself repeatedly was bad enough with Asperger's. It is partly defined by trouble speaking.

You can read more in my 'Why is that lady soo nervous? 'series.

The times I was overwhelmed by how much information I had to give them, I would stutter, leave sentences unfinished and occasionally 'go mute'. I also have a terrible memory when overwhelmed.

## Researching Mental Health Plans

In March 2016 I was once again facing the frustration of having to start explaining everything again from scratch. I was also disappointed by the simplistic mental health plan my GP and I had just made.

In researching what else could be in my plan, I ended up on the Queensland Health's website and its page of guidelines for Doctors.

I was surprised at the list of items that could or should go into one. Many topics I don't remember ever discussing with my past GP's.

I thought this list was a wonderful guideline to use to write my own version. Within two days I had written 8 pages of content.

Eight pages you may say! It wasn't entirely easy. At each step I just picked a few bullet points that I COULD explain. The concept I used was 'what CAN I write about? NOT what SHOULD I write about?

## Immediate Benefits

When I saw a GP a few days later it had been much easier to dress nicely and get on the buses to the clinic. I still wanted to go to the hospital but was also managing my responsibilities better. It was easy to agree with the doctor that I didn't need to go to hospital – that the worst may be over for now.

Instead he reminded me about seeing an established psychologist regularly. I liked this idea and am now seeing a psychologist and a psychiatrist. The latter to get an official diagnosis of Autism Spectrum Disorder. Then I can access other support.

It benefited me with my mental health team referencing parts of the document by speech and flipping pages to find passages. It was affirming. I felt in those moments that they were taking my issues seriously.

In October my Partners in Recovery worker suggested a Residential Program where I could actively work on my goals.

I was settled in and was supported to work on my goals, plan and social life. By the end of the stay I had added another five pages to my plan. That gave me a source of confidence in my writing abilities that continues to this day.

## Unexpected benefits

A few days later I had an Asthma Attack and could barely speak. What I could do was give out my Personal Information page. It was complete with Diagnoses, Medications, health team and emergency contact details.

The ambulance offices and treating emergency team referred to it a few times that night. It was very fortunate that I had that information on hand!

## A source of confidence

Writing my own Mental Health Plan has been affirming, a relief and a source of confidence. Seeing the full Index page with my issues mapped out clearly was both a relief and source of pride. I no longer had to worry about forgetting important facts about my mental health.

If this interests you, I recommend writing your own. The template bullet points I used are at health.gov.au.

Good luck writing your own Mental Health Plan!

# Challenges of writing my own Mental Health Plan

I've previously posted about the benefits of writing my own Mental Health Plan.

You can find the post here. I talked in part about frustration of having to repeat my story to every new professional. I also have trouble speaking and a faulty memory when overwhelmed.

Today I'll write about challenges around writing and having my Mental Health Plan.

*During the writing and revision stage, I referenced content guidelines found on the health.gov.au website. You can view them here.*

## Continuing to work on it

I had to pick a few bullet points at a time to write about. On the first version I disregarded about half of the bullet points.

I knew that I couldn't write on those topics for various reasons – at the time. I was content to leave them be for now, and revise it at a later date.

## Being Over It

There are parts that I skimmed while making revisions. I've kept them because I tried to write as objectively as possible. I imagined myself as a psychiatrist writing a report about a patient.

They may have to be rewritten in the future, but for now I am quite happy with what I've got written down.

## Few actual plans

Being in survival mode, I only had a few things written for my future. They came from my daily To Do list.

What I did write was a very basic crisis management plan. It was warning signs for myself and my sister, as well as a letter to my sister in case I brought myself to hospital one day.

I had to be content with what information was there and knowing that I'd one day research Relapse Prevention Plans.

## Fighting for it

I've had to act very determined to get the revised version put on my GPs records.

I had to be one sided in thought while my body was quailing inside.

In the end she went through it in front of me. She also kept it to get scanned into my file later.

## Feeling my writing was in vain

At times I had to deal with feeling that my doctors weren't taking my writing efforts and issues seriously.

In sessions with my mental health team I *mostly* felt that I had a safety-net. I knew that if I ever had trouble explaining myself, I could direct them to an appropriate part of it.

There were times however when I had the distinct feeling that no one had read it.

Thankfully they have since referenced the document in front of me. To quote from my previous post:

*My mental health team referencing parts of the document by speech and flipping pages to find passages was affirming. I felt in those moments that they were taking my issues seriously.*

Now that I've had enough feedback about it, over time, the plan is a source of confidence. Confidence if I don't explain something accurately and confidence in myself as a hard worker.

Overall, I am very glad that I took the time to write out my own Mental Health Plan. It has been a safeguard in appointments.

Having to search my memory for every answer was something I didn't have to worry about.

If the idea appeals to you, I recommend using this template to write your own Mental Health Plan.

# About the Authors

Karletta Abianac is a blogger, writer, and former public speaker from Queensland, Australia.

As a teenager, she wrote and produced a street zine in Brisbane called Cookies Youth Magazine.
Karletta has long been a community activist; in 2003, she received a Queensland Government Youth Up-Front Award for her "Volunteer Work and Commitment to Social Change", and her first full-length book was entitled Fill in the Gaps - Guide to Community Event Management.

Karletta received an autism diagnosis as an adult, and her memoir series 'I've been there too darl' draws on her life experiences.

In her free time, Karletta enjoys practicing Egyptian hieroglyphs and collecting rocks near her home in Macgregor.

# Contributors

The wonderful contributors to this eBook are:

Lorraine Abbott (Rae)
Kathy Isaacs
Laina Eartharcher (pseudonym)
Liz Marxon (pseudonym)

I thank them again for the care and honesty they showed while writing their stories. You've made my eBook pop and sizzle!

Kathy created Access Health Autism. She supports Autistic people to navigate and access the health system in Australia.

You should view Laina's Silent Wave blog. She has a fantastic way of articulating what being Autistic is like for her.

# Also by Karletta Abianac

## Poetry Collections

Inaccessible: Poetry about inaccessible things.
Hope Emerges: Poetry about hope emerging.

## Memoir Series: I've Been there too, Darl

Successful to Burnt Out: Experiences of Autistic women
Elusive Identity: The Autism spectrum and recreating a sense of identity

## Guides

Fill in the Gaps: Guide to community event management
Elusive Identity: Guide for your values and identity

Printed in Great Britain
by Amazon

78939085R00082